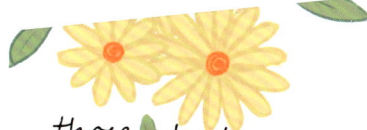

those who hope
in the LORD
will renew their strength
Isaiah 40:31

HEAL
THE SICK

BOOK 1 GIFTS OF A WARRIOR

VALERIE M. QUINATA

God bless you!
Keep Reading!
love, Valerie

Heal the Sick. Gifts of a Warrior. Book 1

Copyright © 2019 by Valerie Quinata

This book is dedicated to my husband and my daughter
Whose love and support
Made everything possible

TABLE OF CONTENTS

1

YOU NEED TO COME WITH ME

I had no pain at all. On a beautiful Saturday in September 2016, I completed my leg of a relay marathon, finishing strong and enjoying my exercise of choice for the last 35 years. The following Wednesday was my annual mammogram appointment. I completed the test and was waiting with another woman to be cleared to leave. She was nervous and shared that she had lost her mother to breast cancer. I told her she was going to be fine, and, a few moments later, a nurse confirmed this and said she could leave. We shared a quick hug before she left, the joy at hearing the results of her test evident on her face. Then the nurse turned to me and said, "You need to come with me." I was struck dumb. I had no pain, no impending sense of doom, my Holy Spirit, Abba Daddy, Jesus; none of them prepped me for this. It was truly a shock.

The next hour passed in a haze of words. I squinted my eyes, trying to comprehend, "found something, need to come back tomorrow, need a biopsy, can you be free, let's get you scheduled…" Coming from a long line of nurses, I recognized what she wasn't saying, "could be nothing, just need to double-check, etc." She knew what she saw, but she couldn't share that; what she could share was a sense of urgency that was authoritative.

From that moment, I was on the treadmill of healthcare procedures that materialize when a cancer diagnosis is first shared. Self-education and an immediate, radical shift of priorities to clear calendars, prepare for treatment, assimilate to the cycle and milestones for 6 chemo treatments, a potential surgery, and possibly up to 5 weeks (are you kidding me, five weeks? Who has time for this?) of radiation, along with all the necessary decisions, conversations, and planning. Within 2 weeks, I had my first chemo down. It was a cyclone of events that, under normal circumstances, would never have been decided so quickly and with so little time to prepare.

As I started my 12-month treatment plan, I felt a peace that was unexplainable. I decided that God would heal me and that good would come from this experience. That I would read, watch, and listen to everything I could find regarding healing. I shared the news with my family and closest friends and met with others to learn, request prayer, receive healing ministrations, and strengthen my resolve to be well. My relationship with God became stronger as I realized all the ways He rescued me, from directing me to the mammogram that saved my life to the daily miracles that solved problems, anticipated needs, comforted me, and ultimately healed me completely. This was not a phase of a typical process for dealing with a life-threatening diagnosis. I wasn't in denial, or angry. I was hunkered down internally, listening intently for the Holy Spirit, checking and double-checking my spirit for clarity and what my next steps should be. Today, I am cancer-free and have no fear that it will return, because the Lord told me what would happen and taught me how to work through this process; it involves confronting the situation, internalizing the healing of Christ, prophesying and daily strengthening in the spirit, knowing how to manage fear, and focusing on purpose and passion. He also said that my purpose would become one of teaching and reaching others to share this information and be the tip of the spear for a new generation of believers who would understand the role that the body of Christ plays in healing.

With all that being said, I was still experiencing the whole course of treatment, and change is difficult. My family and I processed the shock of my entering a complex medical regimen while my 8-year-old daughter began her school year, and during the launch of my new branch at work. The Holy Spirit guided me every day, seeming to stretch minutes for me so I could spend significant time with God each morning. He was a "lamp unto my feet" throughout the process; giving me the understanding and guidance I needed each day through prayer and interacting with Him through scripture, books, and videos.

I will never forget the peace that covered me during that time; how loved and cared for I felt every day. The diagnosis of cancer was not a death sentence; it was a door that opened into an opportunity to experience the love of God in a much deeper way than I had before. It was a series of moments where I faced two paths and had to choose which road to take, but the paths weren't labeled life or death, fight or give up, accept or deny. The paths were labeled, "let God love me through this" or "face this on my own." The outcome of life or death became much less frightening—God had taken the horror out of the situation by switching my focus to Him, not the circumstance.

I want to emphasize this because cancer is a stigma that we've all learned to recoil from; it is modern-day leprosy in that people with the diagnosis are socially quarantined and treated as if they have been cursed. There isn't a clear reason why some die and some survive and this gives way to all sorts of speculation about their lives that have no basis in fact. Because we can't perfectly control the outcome of cancer, many of us mistakenly latch onto characterizations of the patient that cause isolation, judgment, and abandonment. That makes it satan's playground, a place where lies bloom and pain multiplies as individuals struggle to understand something in a world that lacks complete understanding. When we don't understand, we often persecute. This book does not pass judgment on those who have fought cancer in the past, or those who have died after fighting cancer. It is not an attempt at providing a technical understanding of the disease. It is a call to action on behalf of those who are fighting it today because, in many cases, it is our weakness as the body of Christ that places them in that position. It is our weakness because we have been granted authority to heal this disease and we have been stunningly unwilling to do it.

It is a starting point for information to support individuals and families who are in the fight. And it is an invitation to all to entertain the idea that cancer is survivable. The Holy Spirit led me through all of these areas so that I could be healed and share with you—there is much to share and, like Isaiah, there is a fire in my bones to get this information to you quickly.

2
MY CURRICULUM

I felt strongly that I was being taught; that my job was to commit to the same things required of me during school—time, attention, focus, and practice. I made my time with God about listening to Him, submitting to His steps for me. Any free moments were used to watch online healing videos, read books, and study scripture. I would visit my church elders and other local churches. I allowed God to surround me, completely engulf me, through people and words He sent to care for me.

In hindsight, I was able to see the structure of the curriculum shared with me by God. My treatment plan would take a year to complete, and, right before the diagnosis, I lost everything but my immediate family and my relationship with God. Financially, professionally, and personally, I lost so much that a cancer diagnosis should have been a TKO, but God told me that He had other plans for me.

He took me from the most basic topics to very detailed, specific guidance for me alone. In this book, I share all the basics and some of the specifics—each of us must engage with God one-on-one alone through some parts of this journey; my curriculum would not be the same as anyone else's. That is the beauty; the uniqueness and the perfection of a relationship with God. He alone knows exactly what is happening to you, why it is happening, and what you need. Notice I wrote, "what you need" not "what you need to do." This book shares many things that I did, but none of the things I did eclipsed what my Father in heaven did for me. His strongest message to me throughout the illness was always, "Let me love you through this. Let me do this for you." It was more about being than doing. If you are a striver, like me; if you are wired for action, if your circumstances are such that you have little or no trust in others, letting God do something for you can be the toughest thing to learn.

In my case, I can say that being faced with the ultimate threat of death in the form of cancer was the only way I could finally let my guard down and let Him care for me. It was, as Sheldon Vanauken titled his book, a "severe mercy." That key understanding was a specific, personal learning for me, and we all have specific learnings, keys to our freedom, that can only come from doing the work of healing—physically, mentally, emotionally and spiritually—in partnership with God. It is my prayer that you will join me in this.

I also want to stress that some of the deepest work that was accomplished between God and me remains between God and me; I didn't need to share all the details of my weaknesses, shortcomings, and areas of sin that needed to be addressed as part of my healing; God's grace covered that for me. Did I need to face my sins, past and present? Yes, some of them. Were they responsible for my illness and did they require public airing? No. God teaches, He illuminates, forgives and heals; He does not shame, and shame is not part of a healing process. Please know that and release that burden right from the beginning.

If you struggle with whether or not you did something to cause the illness, take a moment to remember a scene from *Goodwill Hunting*—the scene where Robin William's character repeatedly tells Matt Damon's character that it is not his fault – recognize this about your situation, because a cancer diagnosis is not your fault. Shed that thought so you can heal.

I was carried through chapter after chapter of concepts and revelations, advancing in my understanding of God and His will for His children. I developed goals, prayers, patterns of thought and behavior that were all geared toward moving through the healing process and growing in my relationship with God and others. I tracked my miracles, organized my prayers, and applied what I was learning to my life every day.

I now realize that what God was preparing me to do was share all this information with others; with you specifically. You. This book is about what God did for me, and I praise my Abba Daddy for every way He rescued me, but it's also about what God wants to do for *you*. Are you afraid? Frightened out of your mind at times? Are you desperate for help or considering ending your fight in a number of ways? Please read this first. And even if you don't make it through the book, even if you don't make it past this page, know that God loves you. He is not abandoning you, the Kingdom of God is near you. He is as close as your breath. Give Him access to your life and your issues by giving Him your time and attention. He has miracles in store for us all, and that includes you.

There is no limit to what God can do for you, and His requirements are as small as a mustard seed. Consider the least you have to offer Him, the smallest thing you can give to Him. It doesn't matter what it is, as long as you are reaching out for Him, He will be there for you in ways that will comfort, provide for, and help you. Test Him in this now. Offer Him your mustard seed-sized trust, if that's all you have; that's fine. Right now, ask Him to show you something, do something for you, and meet a need that you have. What do you have to lose? I don't know you and you don't know me, but if you have made it this far, I know you can feel the pull of God on your life right now—you are not reading this book by chance. Start your healing process by offering to God what you need and be alert to His answer. That will be the start of your learning, as it was for me.

3

THE GOOD, THE BAD, AND THE MIRACULOUS

The biopsy was painful, and I was given an immediate diagnosis of Stage 2 breast cancer, the specifics of which were aggressive. My first words were, "I've got an 8-year-old daughter and a husband—I can't tap out. I'm the breadwinner, there will be no time off, I can't tap out." But at that moment, I was flooded with peace; a peace that grew stronger over the time it took for me to process my new reality.

Again, the Holy Spirit led me, this time putting up a mental wall every time I succumbed to asking "Why? Why me, God, why?" The question alone seemed to bring a wave of fear, depression, loss, and emptiness that drained me of resolve. Instead, He taught me to run to Him, run to Him like a child, with outstretched arms. I envisioned myself running to Him with the feet of a toddler, running behind Him and into the folds of His robes for protection. From this vantage point, I gathered strength, switched my focus to hope, and rested in Him as my protector.

The greatest psalm of protection is Psalm 91, and I would re-peat it over and over, especially verses 3-7, which I've highlighted below:

Surely he will save you

from the fowler's snare

and from the deadly pestilence.

He will cover you with his feathers,

and under his wings you will find refuge;

his faithfulness will be your shield and rampart.

You will not fear the terror of night,

nor the arrow that flies by day,

nor the pestilence that stalks in the darkness,

nor the plague that destroys at midday.

A thousand may fall at your side,

ten thousand at your right hand,

but it will not come near you.

Here is some scripture art with the same verses. Please feel free to use this, to print it out and post it wherever you will see it regularly; to get it down in your spirit.

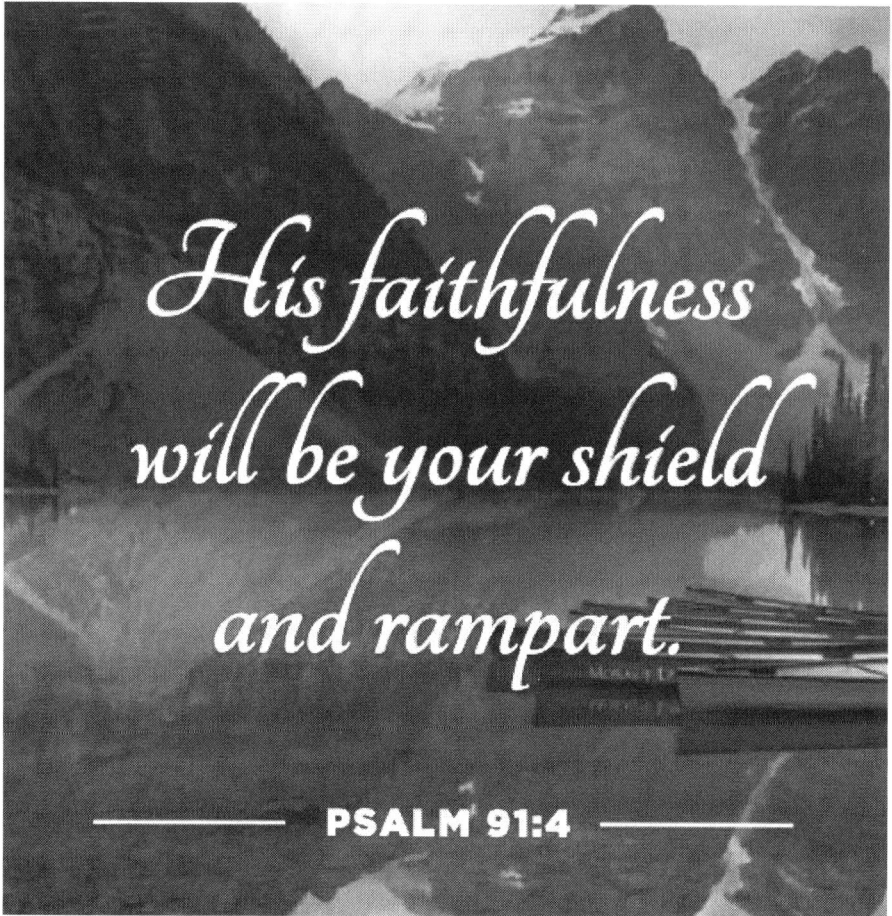

His faithfulness will be your shield and rampart.

PSALM 91:4

This was a lesson about choosing my reality and short-circuiting the tricks of satan. When your thoughts lead to emptiness, loneliness, a seemingly endless void without hope, know that those are not God's thoughts. They are not for you; they are a lie from the father of lies. Learn to switch your thoughts to thoughts of God. The way that works for you will be very personal to you. The Holy Spirit will show you how—just ask. The Bible says it like this: "…whatever is true, whatever is noble, whatever is right, whatever is pure, whatever is lovely, whatever is admirable—if anything is excellent or praiseworthy—think about such things" Philippians 4:8.

It may be through envisioning something like I mentioned about running to Him and hiding in His robes, or it could be as simple as saying, "Nope, no" when satan's thoughts cross your mind. You must realize who the enemy is—but once you've done that, refuse to give him airtime. Cut him off the moment he begins to attack. Use scripture, imagery, or a physical movement like waving your hand, as in, "BYE, satan!" This is an important first step in your healing, linking your thoughts to God, especially when negativity comes. Find scriptures about healing (there are many in this book) and speak those scriptures aloud as often as you can. You are now part of the resistance; you are on the battlefield, and you are fighting.

The activity of shifting your thoughts is foundational to your training. Give priority to this work, the same as you would physical training. The devil will flee because Jesus commands that he must flee if you resist. Want extra credit? When negative thoughts come, turn your thoughts to God and then pray for the healing of all who are fighting cancer. Proverbs 6:31 says that thieves must pay for what they've stolen sevenfold if they are caught—make the devil pay for trying to come after you! Here is an example:

In the name of Jesus Christ of Nazareth, I declare satan has been stealing my peace and my health, along with the health of millions of people fighting cancer. The word of the Lord in Proverbs 6:31 states, "yet if he is caught, he must pay sevenfold, though it costs him all the wealth of his house." I declare satan has been caught and he is now paying me along with everyone that is fighting cancer back sevenfold for everything stolen from us all. Amen.

Dodie Osteen, when diagnosed with Stage IV liver cancer, would stand on her Bible every day, speaking aloud the words of healing within it and stating that she was, literally, standing on His word, His promises. Do what you are led to do to restore power and peace to your mind.

The night after my biopsy, after spending the rest of the day in a robotic state, scheduling follow-up tests, procedures, chemotherapy infusions, and surgery, I asked God to help me. Just help me. If all you can say at this point is one word, make it "Jesus." That's all you need. "Jesus." I would repeat it over and over. I couldn't form any other words. And God gave me a dream. I was in a boat that was just big enough for me and I was on the water; it seemed like I was in a harbor, and the water was a deep, beautiful blue. He spoke to me and said, "This won't be as bad as you think. You've told me you want to live to be over a hundred; this is a tune-up. You will hold your daughter's granddaughter."

Please understand, I do not dream, or I don't remember dreams if I have them. I have not spent my life as a believing adult in a relationship with God that includes prophetic communications. Not me. I'm the one who was always out in front, "helping God," basically making decisions I was sure He would agree with. But despite that weakness, even though I am in no way perfect or a perfect follower of Christ, God knew my heart and He knew I needed Him to show up in a way I would never forget, a way that would carry me through the next 13 months. I made an unformed request based on something I truly needed from Him and He responded. I chose to believe every word He said in that dream. Even now, when I wake up in the night with a feeling of panic, I remind myself of those words and I am calm again.

A key point I've had to learn over and over again is that God doesn't withhold His help, His love, and His guidance until you are "perfect." Because of His Son, you are already perfect and able to ask Him for what you need at any time. Please print this off, post it everywhere, and make it your cellphone wallpaper. You are perfect now, and He is here for you now.

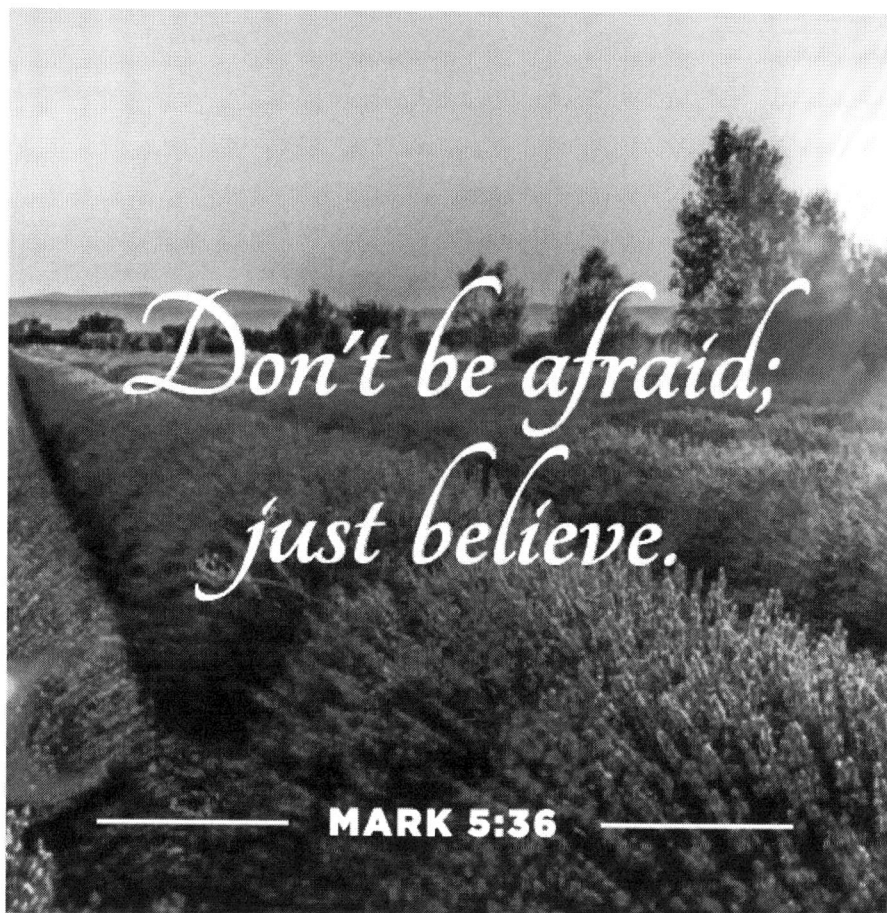

Don't be afraid; just believe.

MARK 5:36

A life-threatening diagnosis means that you must anchor yourself to God; take every thought captive and share it with Him; continually ask Him to help, guide, and protect you. Do it all day, every day. I learned that if I walked around with my headphones on, I could speak to God anywhere, anytime, and those around me just assumed I was on a call. Which I was. I prayed, thanked Him, asked for help, and told Him I needed Him. Then, I listened. I learned that once I spent as much time listening as talking, I began to hear Him more regularly, to the point that we now have conversations, some of which I'll share with you.

The world tells you that it is weak to fully depend on anyone, but God wants to be with you 24/7 if that is what you need. And who needs it more than someone in a significant health crisis? I realized that He didn't just want me to go through this process with Him, He showed me that He would go through it with me; be right there going through it, not hovering above me, not checking in on Sundays. He was experiencing it with me so that I would never be alone. And I never was—ever. It didn't matter if I wasn't in a practical, prayerful attitude, or attending my seventh church service that week, or mailing checks to support others. I didn't need to earn His presence in my life, and neither do you. God will take whatever you have, whenever you have it. Hand over your fears, your problems, your questions, hand them over, throw them off, drop them into a well, light them up in a campfire and watch the embers head into the night sky. It doesn't matter how you do it, but give them to God so He can help you get satan off your back and attend to your needs so you can heal and live the life that was meant for you.

The next step in my treatment plan was preparation; testing to provide a more accurate diagnosis and ensure that I could withstand the intended treatments, including a 45-minute MRI, an echocardiogram, and the surgical insertion of a port, through which I would get my chemotherapy infusions. My first infusion was only 2 weeks out and I needed to complete these procedures before the first infusion. I failed at my first attempt at the MRI. The scan required me to be on my stomach for 45 minutes, and I kept panicking during the procedure so they sent me home with a requirement to get a sedative from my doctor and return the next day.

I had to drive myself to the hospital for the test, so taking the sedative ahead of time was not an option. Instead, I found a healing video by David Baker that took at least 45 minutes, which was miraculous, because I wouldn't be able to move once I was on the table. I listened to it throughout the procedure and was able to complete the test peacefully. I listened to this miraculous video several times throughout my treatment. It laid the foundation for understanding and believing in the healing power that Christ died to provide for us. There is a healing video by David Baker that I listened to repeatedly, in the car, while working, and once during a marathon MRI session. If you are conflicted about doctors, God, or healing, this can help you.

4

GOD'S WILL TO HEAL

With the MRI completed, I focused on preparing myself for the port procedure and chemotherapy. The next phase of my healing curriculum was to establish in my mind that God wanted to heal me, that He had provided for it through His son, Jesus, and that He wanted it for me specifically by reaching me personally through my dream. I tracked every verse that proved God's will is to heal His children and read them aloud every day. Every day. I chose to believe that I could be healed. That was the start. I've included many of these verses for you here, but I encourage you to search them out for yourself. God will make it clear which are most important to you. In the back of the book I have include scripture art for many of these scriptures. Please use them!

First, I had to understand the extent of God's power and that He included me and all believers in the scope of it. Paul makes this clear in Ephesians 1:17-23, so I read these words every day:

I keep asking God, the glorious Father of our Lord Jesus Christ, to give you spiritual wisdom and insight so that you might grow in your knowledge of God. I pray that your hearts will be flooded with light so that you can understand the confident hope he has given to those he called—his holy people who are his rich and glorious inheritance. I also pray that you will understand the incredible greatness of God's power for us who believe him. This is the same mighty power that raised Christ from the dead and seated him in the place of honor at God's right hand in the heavenly realms. Now he is far above any ruler or authority or power or leader or anything else—not only in this world but also in the world to come. God has put all things under the authority of Christ and has made him head over all things for the benefit of the church. And the church is his body; it is made full and complete by Christ, who fills all things everywhere with himself.

Paul's words included those he was communicating with at the time, but it also includes you and me, his body, which is the church. And he speaks about the power that is the highest, a power that was available to him then but is also available to us now and throughout our eternal lives.

These words made it clear to me that, as a believer, I am part of the body of Christ and I have available to me the same power that raised Jesus from the dead, and that power is available to me now, today, and forever. Always. All ways. All power. The source of and connection to this power is Jesus. When I was learning this, it helped to have a visual image that depicted God's power and my role in the body of Christ. I felt like a young person, sometimes a little girl, at times a young woman, surrounded by the beauty and force of God, and I searched for pictures that aligned with that in my spirit and put them where I could see them as I studied.

The process of finding pictures that identified my unique position was a healing process itself, and it helped me become aligned with God. One of the pictures I chose was of my mother and grandfather. My mom was about 5 and she was spending time with her dad on a rowboat in one of the lakes in Washington State in Fort Lewis, where he was stationed. He looks protective and powerful, and my mother is happy and laughing, safe between his powerful arms as he rowed the boat. I always get a sense of protection and journey from this picture – it enabled me to connect with God about where we were going and feel safe throughout the journey.

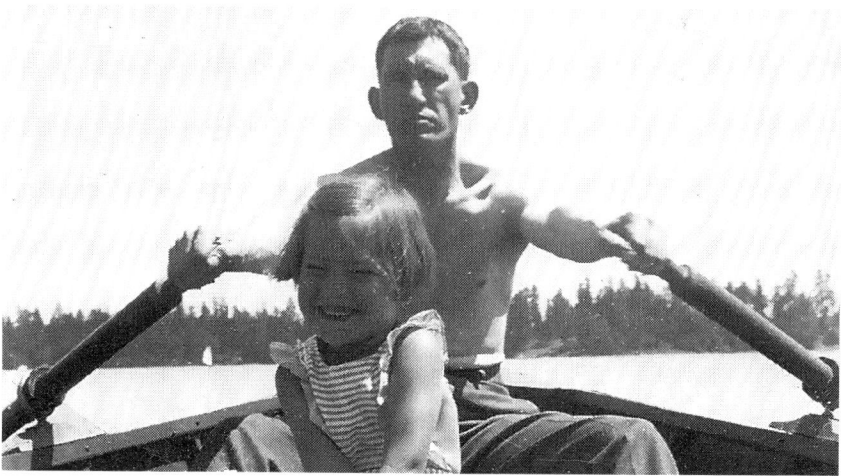

This knowledge was my foundation for learning, the rock upon which my healing was based.

As I continued to study scriptures on healing, I learned that Jesus was a studier of the holy scriptures that were available to Him during His time on earth. His Father had provided scripture on healing that was both appropriate for the time it was written as well as prophetically charged to be effective in the future. He would have read the same words we can read about healing, from the first books of the Bible to Psalms to the prophets. And in His lifetime, Jesus provided anointed healing that would be noted in the New Testament through to Revelations. Take your time with these scriptures about healing; write down for yourself those scriptures that resonate with you; read them all every day and focus on one or two each week; make them a part of your life during this time so God's power can work on you through them.

OLD TESTAMENT

"You intended to harm me, but God intended it for good; to accomplish what is now being done, the saving of many lives." Genesis 50:20

"If you listen carefully to the Lord your God and do what is right in his eyes, if you pay attention to his commands and keep all his decrees, I will not bring on you any of the diseases I brought on the Egyptians, for I am the Lord, who heals you." Exodus 15:26

"Worship the Lord your God, and his blessing will be on your food and water. I will take away sickness from among you, and none will miscarry or be barren in your land. I will give you a full life span." Exodus 23:25-26

MAJOR PROPHETS

"But he was pierced for our transgressions,

he was crushed for our iniquities;

the punishment that brought us peace was on him,

and by his wounds we are healed."

Isaiah 53:5

"I will make peace your governor and well being your ruler."

Isaiah 60:17

MINOR PROPHETS

"Come, let us return to the Lord.

He has torn us to pieces

but he will heal us;

he has injured us

but he will bind up our wounds.

After two days he will revive us;

on the third day he will restore us,

that we may live in his presence."

Hosea 6:1-2

"I will repay you for the years the locusts have eaten—
the great locust and the young locust,
the other locusts and the locust swarm—
my great army that I sent among you.
You will have plenty to eat, until you are full,
and you will praise the name of the Lord your God,
who has worked wonders for you;
never again will my people be shamed.
Then you will know that I am in Israel,
that I am the Lord your God,
and that there is no other;
never again will my people be shamed." Joel 2:25-27

PSALMS

"Lord my God, I called to you for help,
and you healed me." Psalm 30:2

"Surely he will save you
from the fowler's snare
and from the deadly pestilence.
He will cover you with his feathers,
and under his wings you will find refuge;
his faithfulness will be your shield and rampart.
You will not fear the terror of night,

nor the arrow that flies by day,

nor the pestilence that stalks in the darkness,

nor the plague that destroys at midday.

A thousand may fall at your side,

ten thousand at your right hand,

but it will not come near you."

Psalm 91:3-7

Praise the Lord, my soul,

and forget not all his benefits—

who forgives all your sins

and heals all your diseases,

who redeems your life from the pit

and crowns you with love and compassion,

who satisfies your desires with good things

so that your youth is renewed like the eagle's."

Psalm 103:2-5

"He allowed no one to oppress them; for their sake
He rebuked kings. Do not touch my anointed ones;
and do my prophets no harm." Psalm 105:14-15

"Then He brought them out with silver and gold, and
among His tribes there was not one who stumbled."
Psalm 105:37

"Then they cried to the Lord in their trouble,

and he saved them from their distress.

He sent out his word and healed them;

he rescued them from the grave.

Let them give thanks to the Lord for his unfailing love

and his wonderful deeds for mankind."

Psalm 107:19-21

"I shall not die but live and declare the works of the Lord." Psalm 118:7

NEW TESTAMENT

"Jesus called his twelve disciples to him and gave them authority to drive out impure spirits and to heal every disease and sickness." Matthew 10:1

"When Jesus had called the Twelve together, he gave them power and authority to drive out all demons and to cure diseases." Luke 9:1

"Heal the sick who are there and tell them, 'The kingdom of God has come near to you.'" Luke 10:9

"The seventy-two returned with joy and said, "Lord, even the demons submit to us in your name." Luke 10:17

"I have given you authority to trample on snakes and scorpions and to overcome all the power of the enemy; nothing will harm you." Luke 10:19

"For whosoever shall call upon the name of the Lord shall be saved." Romans 10:13

"Is any one of you sick? He should call the elders of the church to pray over him and anoint him with oil in the name of the Lord." James 5:14

"I know the one in whom I trust, and I am sure that he is able to guard what I have entrusted to him until the day of his return...[and] being confident of this, that he who began a good work in me will carry it on to completion until the day of Christ Jesus." 2:Timothy 1:12, Phillipians 1:6

I was overwhelmed by the evidence of God's healing grace throughout written history, from Genesis to Revelations, where John foretells about healing in his vision of Revelations 2:22:

"On each side of the river stood the tree of life, bearing twelve crops of fruit, yielding its fruit every month. And the leaves of the tree are for the healing of the nations."

Remember when I wrote that as you spend more time listening, God will speak to you more? This was one of those moments. When it dawned on me the provision God made for healing throughout time, He said to me, "So why would anyone think I've stopped? Why would I go against my Word and stop healing?"

I've never felt comfortable with prayers where people ask God to heal, "if it is His will." That feels passive aggressive and as if I'm shirking my duty as a Christian. Jesus didn't die so we could double check with Him to make sure it was ok to heal somebody and then set Him up for the failure if it didn't happen. That isn't how he did things. He may have stopped to align His spirit with His Father about how to heal, but not about whether or not He had permission to do it. Remember the scene in the synagogue where he healed the man with the shriveled hand? He was expressly going against the culture of the day and the understanding of the religious requirements of the Jewish leaders. In His words in Luke 6:9, Jesus said to them, "I ask you, which is lawful on the Sabbath: to do good or to do evil, to save life or to destroy it?" For me, the question about whether or not God wills to heal us is answered, unequivocally in the affirmative. Yes, He wills to heal us.

He had a mission and a purpose that drove Him, that kept Him aligned with His Father that was aided by the Holy Spirit. In John 10:18 He says, "No one takes it (my life) from me, but I lay it down of my own accord. I have authority to lay it down and authority to take it up again. This command I received from my Father." I took this as a command for me as well and determined that I have some say in whether I die or not, that I have some power to wield in that decision. So I created a prayer to affirm this:

Jesus said, "No one takes it (my life) from me, but I lay it down of my own accord. I have authority to lay it down and authority to take it up again. This command I received from my Father." I take this as a command for me as well, and I declare now that I do not now and never will lay my life down for cancer, cancer treatments, or side effects of cancer. I will not lay my life down for any accidents, illness, injury, sickness or disease. I will not lay my life down for any attacks or demons coming against me. I do not lay my life down for another 60 years at least. And should Jesus, my Jesus, return during that time, I will be able to answer YES when He asks, "Is there still faith on the earth?" Amen. I repeated this every day and built my faith for the power of Christ to heal me.

5

YOU WILL DO GREATER THINGS

Now that I could clearly see God's provision for healing through His Word, it was time for me to strengthen my belief by maturing my understanding of Christ's work on the cross as a way to be healed. Each morning, I would complete my devotions, speaking aloud the verses on healing that I had written down on previous days. Then I would turn to scriptures where healing was mentioned and add more to my list.

I knew that Jesus taught his disciples how to heal and charged them with healing everyone they came near. He said in John 14:12: Very truly I tell you, whoever believes in me will do the works I have been doing, and they will do even greater things than these because I am going to the Father. So, I reasoned, if Christ healed everyone He encountered, and I am supposed to do greater things than that, if all believers are supposed to do greater things than that, let's start doing them!

I understood this verse to set an expectation for the body of Christ to believe in Him and to do something, whether I did the same as Him or greater than Him, just DO THINGS, as He did while He walked the earth. The path to restoring healing to the body of Christ involves learning, believing and doing. Our source for healing is Christ and His sacrifice on the cross. Isaiah 53:5 tells us: He was wounded for our transgressions; He was crushed for our iniquities; the chastening for our wellbeing fell upon Him, and by His wounds we are healed. This was a central concept, so I made scripture art to study it in another way. Feel free to print the scripture art below and put it somewhere where you see it every day. Or make it wallpaper for your cell phone or computer, whatever it takes to get this understanding down in your spirit, do it. By His wounds I am healed; I would repeat this over and over every day, readying myself for treatments and preparing my mind, as much as possible, for the battles to come.

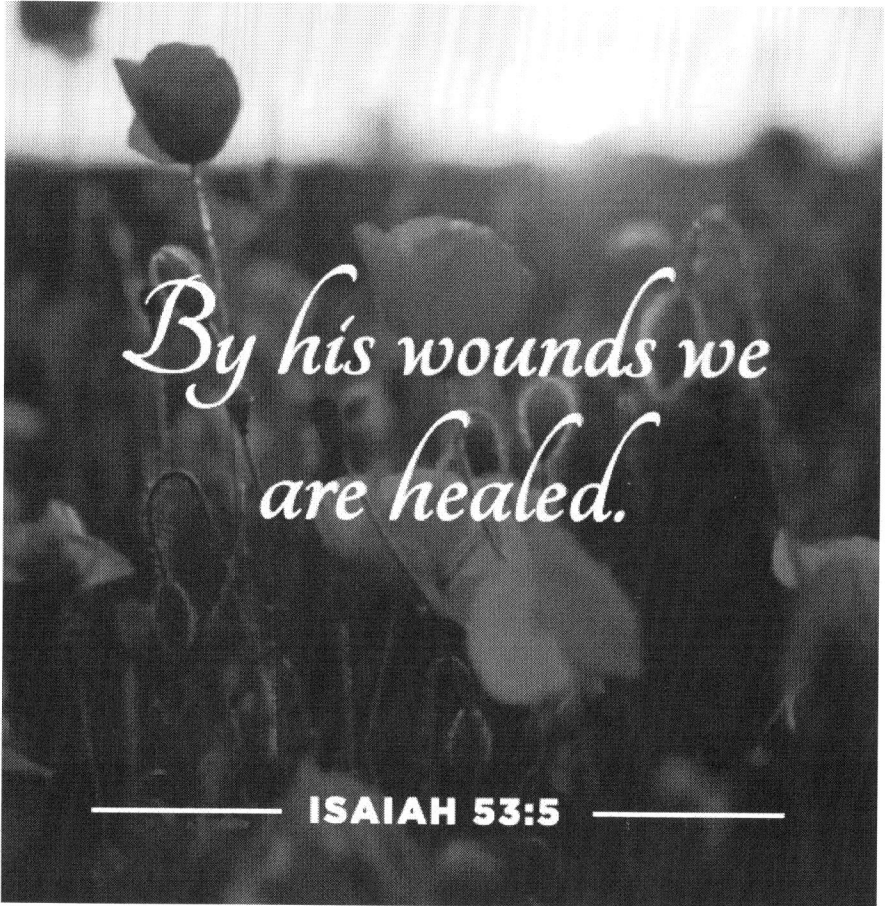

By his wounds we are healed.

ISAIAH 53:5

When Jesus died on the cross for us, He took all illness, accidents, injuries, diseases and sickness, even diseases and sickness that we didn't know about at the time, and He bore them on the cross, giving us victory over them. He granted authority to all who believed in Him to heal and showed His disciples how to do it, as shared in Matthew 10:1: Jesus called his 12 disciples to Him and gave them authority to drive out impure spirits and to heal every disease and sickness.

He then told His disciples to share these healing gifts with others, in Luke 10:9: Heal the sick who are there and tell them, "The kingdom of God has come near to you," and in Matthew 10:7-8: As you go, proclaim this message: "The kingdom of heaven has come near." Heal the sick, raise the dead, cleanse those who have leprosy, drive out demons. Freely you have received; freely give.

The body of Christ is equipped and has been told to heal. For many years, these gifts have only been practiced sparingly, but that doesn't limit the gift or alter God's will for healing to occur. I read several authors who shared their experiences of learning to heal. Alice Cresswell's *A Diary of Miracles*, *The Praying Medic's Divine Healing Made Simple*, and Bill Johnson and Randy Clark's *Essential Guide to Healing* were so compelling that by the time I finished reading them, I couldn't understand why every Christian wasn't healing everybody all the time. With information like this available to us, how are we not all doing this? That's when I learned that many denominations, including my own, did not consider healing in the name of Jesus to be a legitimate Christian activity.

Given my situation, I chose not to be deterred by Christians who wanted to discuss whether or not Jesus intended us to heal each other in His name. I considered that discussion a luxury to be had by unaffected, vibrant, and healthy people, while I identified with the man in the synagogue who had a shriveled hand, who needed a new hand regardless of the day of the week or location that healing took place.

I had studied scripture myself and it was clear to me that Jesus called us to heal the sick. The fact that the body of Christ was divided at all on this point seemed to me to be fraught with confusion, arrogance, ignorance of scripture and the hubris of tradition. But, the result—the death of the innocent, deaths by the millions, along with the greed involved in billions of dollars in healthcare fees—who else could be behind this hypocrisy, this contempt for compassion but satan? Who else could deceive generations of people, successfully recreating over and over again the scene in the synagogue where religious leaders attempt to stop Jesus from healing someone? I chose to believe I was healed and that I could also heal, that it was my duty to heal in the name of Jesus as the Holy Spirit directs me.

I mustered my courage to pray for strangers, to pray for acquaintances, to pray in their presence and to pray at a distance—all things Jesus, my Jesus, did in His lifetime and granted me the authority to do when He died for me. I believed in healing in Jesus's mighty name and applied it in my life every day. I have to add that this behavior, inquiring after strangers in the airport, or on a bus, or a Facebook post, whether or not I could pray for their healing, was not in my usual repertoire of conversation. It was and still is a slightly weird thing to do, but I've never had someone turn me down. Praying for others strengthened me and brought me peace as I continued with my treatments.

I passed the echocardiogram without incident and was scheduled for the port outplacement surgery two days before my first infusion. I took each of these tests either at the end of the day after work or during my lunch, but the port placement involved general anesthesia and I had to miss half a day. It was time to share with others what my situation was, and I struggled with how to refer to the illness.

God never allowed me to say or write the words "I have cancer" or that "I received a diagnosis of cancer." The words were unable to form in my mouth. I said that I had been given a diagnosis of cancer, and I rarely even said that. He shut my lips when it came to owning the disease; I treated it as a temporary situation that didn't exist in the spiritual me.

The Holy Spirit showed me that our words are powerful and must be used to support us. None of us is owned by illness, and, technically, we are not cancer survivors. In fact, by the power of God Almighty, cancer did not survive me. That makes me a conqueror, not a survivor! I spoke that truth out every day, all day long. I created artwork with that saying, which you can freely use.

By the power of God,
Cancer did not survive me.

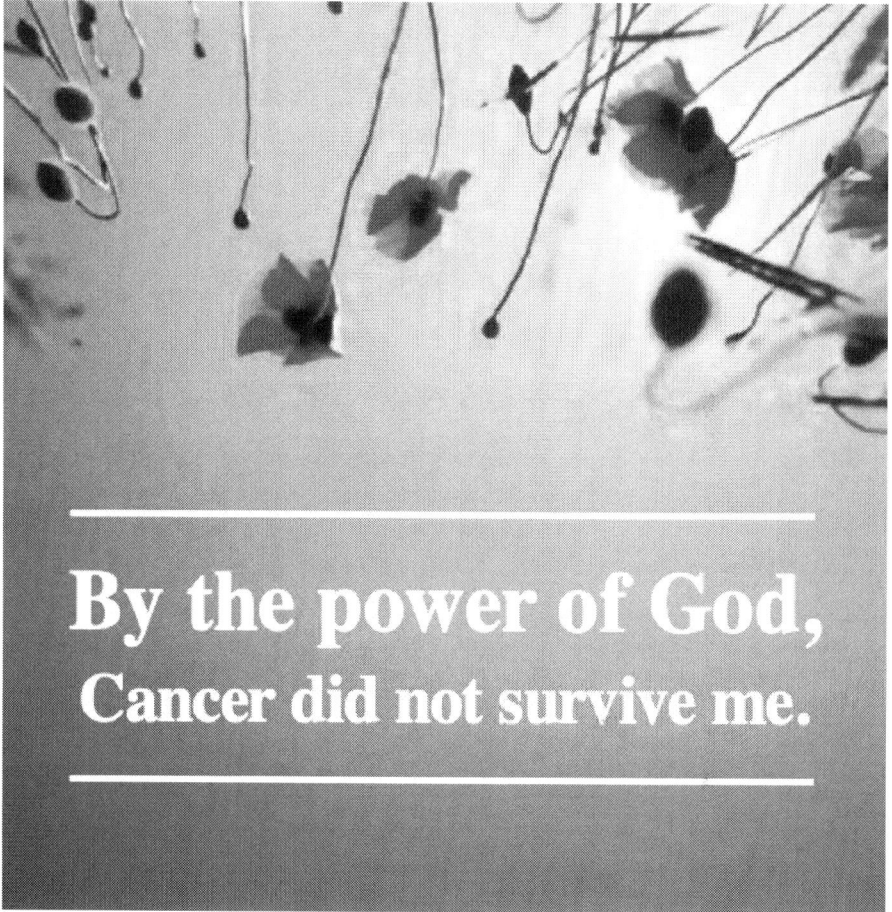

I decided to say that I had been given a diagnosis of breast cancer and that it was stage 2 which meant I could work successfully throughout treatment. For the most part, I was met with encouragement, support, and the promise of prayers. There were some who I refer to as pallbearers—by their words, it was clear that in their minds, I was already in the box. I identified them quickly and spent no time on them or with them. I rarely spoke about my situation or the illness, as I considered myself healed and spoke about that instead.

I rarely asked people for their prayers because I found some who misunderstood God's will and Jesus's plan for healing and would pray things like, "If it's God's will, please heal…" As I wrote earlier, this type of prayer does not fully draw upon our power and capability as Christians. Instead, I asked people to stand and agree with me in prayer regarding my complete healing by Jesus's work on the cross. We don't need to ask God to heal us; He has already told us that it is His will. Instead, we outline the healing that needs to take place and thank Him and Jesus for it. To ask God for less than He is capable of doing is passive-aggressive—we must be honest about what we need. He already knows what we need, anyway; what He is looking for is faith, faith that He exists, that He knows our needs, that we will be honest with Him and that we expect big things from Him!

I completed the port placement, impressed by the accomplishments that have been made in the medical industry as I readied myself for the first infusion. The toxicity of chemotherapy drugs wrecks the veins that carry them, so the port is used to allow the drugs access to the body through larger veins that have a better chance at withstanding the toxins. I worked in my daily devotions to develop a plan for healing and protecting my veins along with the rest of my body when chemo started. I prayed that no part of my body would be affected by either cancer, cancer treatments, and surgeries; that Christ, who makes all things new, was already there, protecting my bodily systems, renewing them so that they all operated as God intended them. I pursued peace for my body throughout the procedures with prayer. Here is an example of a prayer that you can use:

In the name of the Lord Jesus Christ of Nazareth, I declare that all cancer, side effects from cancer, cancer treatments, and surgeries leave me now; that Jesus Himself is restoring my body and that it now operates as God intended it. By the power of Jesus, who took all sickness and disease with Him to the cross and left it there, I declare I am healed of cancer, all cancer side effects, and all fear and anxiety.

In Christ Jesus, who makes all things new, I declare that all the cells in my body are aligning with the Word of God and operating as they were originally designed. I command all the cells in my body that were negatively impacted by cancer, cancer side effects, fear and anxiety to line up with God's Truth that I am fearfully and wonderfully made. Holy Spirit, please destroy all cells that refuse to change to accept God's Truth. I speak to every generation of cells in my body and call forth the creation of new, strong, powerful and healthy cells. I bless them with the abundant life of the Lord Jesus Christ! Thank you, Father!

6

PREPARING FOR CHEMO

The weekend before my first infusion, I created a Facebook page for my thoughts and experiences as well as the daily miracles, encouragements, and lessons I learned. There is no way to prepare for chemo; you've heard it's bad, you know it's going to make you physically sick, but until it happens, you feel fine. I spent time playing with my daughter and ate dinner with my family. I cut and donated my hair. I was on a steroid cocktail so I wasn't sleeping but my prayer life was so strong that I spent the time awake studying. In the beginning, I wrote prayers. One of my first prayers after being given the diagnosis was about prophesying healing over my life. I prophesied healing over my life and my body. Every. Single. Day. I encourage you to use the prayer below to develop a prophetic prayer for your healing:

Father, I know You are prophesying over my life now and I add to this prophecy my thanks and gratitude to You for the blessings You have poured out on my life, even though others looking at my life right now might think the opposite. My testimony doesn't come from the final victory alone, it also comes from the faith that allowed me to stand when everything was coming against me. It comes from the incredible experience of being loved by You through a difficult situation and being introduced to people that You sent to surround me so that I would know Your care during this frightening, looking-death-in-the-eye season. I will forever be grateful for the closeness we share right now. In the name of Jesus Christ of Nazareth, I declare healing over my body; I declare that I am completely healed from cancer, cancer treatments, and surgeries. My body is operating in love, in the fullness of Christ, and as God intended it. In Jesus's name, Amen.

There are more prayers and examples of prayers at the end of the book. Please use them, make them your own, post and share them with others who need them.

I continued to listen to every podcast, watch every video and read every book I could find about healing. Every positive message, blessing, prophetic word, and story about the healings of others became a blanket and a shield for me, a woven garment of protection that altered my reality and enabled me to block out anything negative. In Dodie Osteen's words, "…Deny that cancer or illness is changing your life." There is also a Joel Osteen video that I drew strength from as I readied myself for battle, titled "Don't Waste Your Pain," which I watched/listened to repeatedly.

The Holy Spirit showed me that I needed to get into the presence of God in every way I could—memes, spiritual books, sermons, music, and worship at my church or online, visits to holy places, and, most importantly, time alone with Him. This wasn't difficult for me then because I was on a steroid cocktail to counteract nausea from the chemo and didn't sleep much. My relationship with God was as regular as a heartbeat, humbling in nature, and I was completely open to Him. When you need Him, when you must learn to live, when you decide to open yourself to His teachings, an amazing adventure begins.

I would distill my learning down to a single word or phrase and make a painting or a full-page sketch of it in my daily calendar, reminding myself over and over again to speak it out loud and get it down into my spirit. I've included many of them in this book, and you are free to copy them and use them yourself; in fact, please consider doing so. I believe it will help you in your healing.

While I have not had a near-death experience, I have had a look-death-in-the-face experience, and, similar to the way people with near-death experiences describe it, the peace of God was there for me immediately. I was not afraid. My sense was one of being held; the safety net was in place, "no harm would come near my tent" Psalm 91:10. But a significant part of my shield was being in the presence of God always, as often as I could be. The presence of God was a four-cornered, glowing net that could draw me up and away from fear, attacks from the world and attacks from within. To maintain the net required the presence of God and a desire to be close to Him became the highest priority of my life.

I continued my study of healing and embraced God's word, His presence, His saints, and all manner of healers who worked in the name of Jesus. I filled my mind with every kind of positive, Christ-filled energy, from music to prayers to spoken and written words, to holy places. Everywhere I looked, there was Jesus, hand outstretched, pulling me out of the deep water with a patient confidence that I would learn something, that I was precious and loved beyond my understanding.

7

WE ARE MEANT TO BE WELL

God's word and His actions throughout history have displayed that our bodies, our physical shells, are capable of wholeness, wellness, and healing; not made to be worn out or injured or pursued by sickness. Adam, Eve and the patriarchs of the Bible lived hundreds of years, and in Deuteronomy 29:5, the Lord says, "During the forty years that I led you through the wilderness, your clothes did not wear out, nor did the sandals on your feet." Jesus ministered healing as a foundational act during His time on earth, and in Acts 5:15, we learned that His apostles' shadows could heal!

God made a perfect plan for all to be healed. As Christians, bearing the mantle of the covenant between God and Abraham, we have the power of God, through the Holy Spirit, manifested by Christ's work on the cross, to cast out infirmity, illness, demonic forces and anything coming against us; to live outside of this capability is to live beneath our covenant rights as children of Abraham.

But it takes learning, accepting, receiving and redemptive work for everything I just said to take hold in your life, especially if you need it to manifest and manifest pronto, which was my case. So mine was a crash course in growth as a Christian. I read His word daily along with every Christian author I could find who wrote about healing. I watched videos and listened to healing messages. I attended healing services, including the powerful work of healing worship. And I learned that many, many people are walking among us that have healed completely from cancer. It is in no way a death sentence, yet the overwhelming darkness that surrounds it is very hard to break through for individuals without the power of Jesus.

It's time to shine a light in the darkness and declare victory over cancer and all forms of illness as we grow in our understanding and capability to heal others and ourselves. There is a great call for Christians to manifest this skill. I refer to it as a skill versus a gift because every Christian can and is supposed to heal themselves and others. Christ gave us the blueprint time after time, with every healing act. In Luke 10:19 He says, "I have given you authority…nothing will harm you." This is more than reassurance, it is a call to action, and it was what He said to His disciples before they left to minister to others. It is time to continue to evolve this skill throughout the body of Christ.

There are keys to the use of this skill and there are training requirements. Along with belief, the ability to heal requires openness, sensitivity, maturity, and emotional strength. These all need to be developed, along with practice. That's right, practice. Every Christian healer I studied went through a process of healing where nothing happened. People weren't healed. It was embarrassing; heartbreaking for those they were trying to help and a strong deterrent to trying again. But they did try again and again until finally, it worked, and once it worked, there was very little that could hold them back.

8

DO NOT FEAR AND DO NOT REBEL

These words hit me powerfully as my studies began and set the tone for my "curriculum" from the Holy Spirit after that. I would be guided to a topic and a single element of the topic became a key learning that I would review, both in various forms of content and by just repeating the phrase itself. Each section the Holy Spirit covered with me took about two weeks but could take longer if the topic was something that had developed into a stronghold in my mind.

By now I knew that God wanted to heal me and that I wanted to be healed. That I needed to cut off negative thoughts before they took root in my mind. This all made sense, except that the world was somehow weirdly eager to walk out a death sentence with me when it came to cancer because they were so afraid of it. Do not fear and do not rebel. The simplicity of the command got through to me. I didn't need to fight fear as much as I simply needed to obey the command *not to fear*. To jump on that very first synapse of activity that would normally move me into a state of fear and redirect it immediately to the booming sound of God saying DO NOT FEAR AND DO NOT REBEL.

It was like boot camp in the beginning, and I did as the word said without delving into it, but as the practice of jumping in front of the fear synapse with a vision of God booming His command became automatic, I realized the absolute, stark, wholly encompassing NOTHING that fear is. Fear is nothing, it is a lie. Do not fear and do not rebel. There was a reason that this was the first thing the Holy Spirit taught me. It was the first phrase that I journaled over and over, every day throughout my workday, in notebooks, in memes I would construct while doodling on a sticky note. Allowing fear into my mind then became equated with rebellion, with an act of allowing it into my mind. Looked at that way, fear became reduced to a bad habit, like biting my nails or chewing my lip. That's all it was, a bad habit that I allowed to influence me, but I could choose not to do that. I could choose to ignore fear and take all of its power away, making space for the higher power of supernatural problem solving, like healing.

Fear is also a time/space trick of the devil. There are relatively few moments when fear is warranted, compared to the gazillion hours we spend being afraid. Fear can do nothing outside of the actual moment when it is warranted, and what it does in that nanosecond is alert us to call out to God. Every other moment I spent afraid was a complete illusion because the reality was that during those other moments, I was alive, breathing, loving and being loved. Being afraid would only give the devil a chance to steal my time on earth being loved and replace it with time spent on earth being afraid; now who wants that? I would picture myself outside of my favorite ice cream stand, eating a single scoop of double chocolate with peanut butter ripple, while someone tried to hand me a big, rippling centipede. I would recoil from the insect, of course, and continue eating my ice cream, which was right there in my hand already. Treat fear the same way. Give it right back to satan and hang onto your ice cream; live in the love you have in your life right now. Stay in the moment and deny anyone the ability to move you into an illusion of fear.

My family and I all had to understand this message, and ultimately, we did. So satan, You tried to take so much from my family and me. Among other things, you tried to steal our peace through fear. But grace means that I knew that when my husband was angry over something small or when my daughter needed to be consoled over a nothing knee scrape, they were really afraid for me. They were processing 24/7 fear for me. But that stopped when I stopped being afraid; when I returned to my "normal" self, who laughed and joked and participated in their lives again. And in the name of Jesus Christ of Nazareth whom I serve, I declare you caught, devil, and I'm adding my family's peace to the list of things you are trying to steal but can't. And I hold you accountable through the word of God, Proverbs 6:31: But when he is found, he must repay sevenfold; He must give all the substance of his house.

Devil, you are caught, and I declare my demands for payment now, in Jesus's name, Amen.

9

NEW PRIORITIES

By the grace of God and the power of Jesus, I worked full time during my treatments. I did this because I had to, there was not a choice, but I quickly realized that the more I lived my life as if I was completely healthy, the better I felt. Work allowed me to deny any focus on illness while still caring for myself. I was unable to travel during chemo treatments, and my strength training was put on hold, but those were the only major concessions made.

I learned to wage war against germ invasions in my world, which I boiled down to four major items: cell phones, TV remotes, light switches, and hand towels. I policed these items like a warden and 70/30 alcohol dilution in a spray bottle was my BFF; I became a clean freak about them and I still shrink back from hand towels and anything with a screen that has been in my daughter's possession.

As I waited for my first chemo infusion, my daily patterns emerged with new priorities. Time in the early morning spent studying healing, taking notes and logging on my Facebook page, followed by caring for my family and doing my job. Most days I could accomplish all three. My prayer life became something that operated 24/7 and, as I sought Him, my God, my Abba Daddy filled me with peace, covered me with grace and supplied everything we needed. That sounds warm and fuzzy, but anyone who has gone through cancer treatments or lived with someone who has knows the effort it takes to live normally.

Cancer had a way of acting like a grey filter over everything. I lived my life as if I was normal, but the diagnosis kept threatening to change things without my permission. When I felt it like the sword of Damocles, I remembered that I needed to be there for my family as much as they needed to be there for me. I never talked about our situation with my daughter unless she brought it up; it mattered very little what I said to her during that time. What mattered was that I still showed up for her.Dinnertime was family time, so I resolved that no matter how I felt, I would join them for dinner. Sitting at the table, talking about our day and finding things to be interested in and laugh about, looking my daughter in the eye with every bit of focused attention I could provide; those were the times that would keep us whole and keep fear out of the picture. I prayed to turn the sword into a cross, into a baseball bat, into a smarmy hands-shaping heart through which the sunset prismed out. Anything to boomerang fear back where it came from, while I made dinner, did the laundry, packed a lunch. Maintaining routine was my resistance against fear when it came to my family.

10
DAILY MIRACLES

And the miracles came daily. I can't tell you loudly enough how many miracles surround you right now. They are there, waiting for you. Simple things like critical appointments that went awry. I went to the wrong hospital to get my port surgically placed, and without the port, my chemo sessions couldn't start and they had already been scheduled out four months with surgery immediately afterward; it was a potential tsunami of calendar rework. But oh, hang on, we have an operating room that has that equipment and a doctor who is available today. You're lucky, we can get you right in! Over and over others congratulated me on my "luck" which was never luck at all but blessing after blessing. My situation caused me to walk so closely with God that His blessings chased me down and the more I recognized and thanked Him, the more came for me and my family. God isn't a vending machine, but, as Scott Hamilton points out, attitude is everything:

"This brain tumor has given me a lot more than it has taken away. There are no accidents. Worry will not add one hour to my life, as it says in the Good Book. I want to love every minute of my life. I'm not going to allow anything to throw me off. Through a strong relationship with Jesus, you can endure anything. The only true disability in life is a bad attitude. God is there to guide you through the tough spots. God is there every single time. Every single time." – Scott Hamilton

Just before chemo #1, The Holy Spirit showed me the future during one of my morning studies about blessings, that we are the Sky Net generation, and just like the nuclear attack scenes in the *Terminator* movies, our generation's sense of the future is based on frameworks of end times, wars, catastrophes, death, all the wages of sin. Images flew through my mind of explosions, fire, earthquakes, and tsunamis. But in Romans 5:20, the Bible clearly states that where sin abounds, *grace abounds all the more.* So somewhere in the world, amazing things are happening that more than offset the bad. My job was to find them and spread the news; to keep hope burning for Zion.

There is a coming generation, and we are the tip of that spear, a coming generation that will be part of a spiral UP, not a spiral down. We will believe a new framework for the future, one that says that Sky Net is not the only thing that's going to be happening during the end times. There will also be incredible believing bodies of Christ doing His work, Zion will exist. Think about it. How awesome would the works of grace have to be to accomplish greater than the wages of sin during the end times? Manifest on an awesome scale would be the works of miracles, healings, and harvests for Christ. What types of positive events will be more powerful than earthquakes, tsunamis, and nuclear explosions?

From that perspective, healing me of a little stage 2 breast cancer was easy peasy. Looked at from the vantage point of Zion, an incredible power, the power of Christ, living in me, living in all believers, should make the manifestation of cancer impossible, so why is it here?

When the darkness appears real and is capable of manifesting in our world, there are foundational lies at work. Satan is a liar and the father of lies. I realized that the cancer cells at work in me were not necessarily my enemy, they were a part of me that believed a lie on a cellular level. I found myself talking to them and saying, "I see your energy, your desire to grow, to create. But what you don't realize is that you are destroying me, and once I'm gone, you will be, too. Did someone tell you that by growing faster and faster and taking over my body you would win somehow? Because you won't. Satan is lying when he tells you there is some end game here for you. The very second you grow beyond my capacity to live, you will die. That's how satan works, the ultimate lose/lose, and he will enjoy the trick he played on you. Because without me, you won't exist."

At that moment, I imagined a switch inside me turning off; the stir-crazy cell expression winding down like a jet engine slowing to full stop at the micro-level. A nanosecond of cellular intelligence went, "wait, what?" and kicked the grow crazy switch off.

11
PEACE OVER CONTROL

The day before my first chemo infusion, my port was deciding whether or not it would remain in my body. I needed it to survive the constant IVs, blood draws, infusions, blah blah blah. But I could feel it moving around and causing low-level pain. I was inhabited by something I wanted to be rid of.

I started feeling panicky, checking my temperature, calling my doctor. Two things happened. I spoke with a nurse and God spoke to me. You already know I'm from a family of nurses. I have a picture of my great grandmother in a nursing uniform from the early 1900s. There is a palm tree behind her, because she's in Florida, where it's at least 80 degrees. She is wearing all black and covered in it from head to toe. Just another reason I say that nurses are ministering angels, because she looked purposeful and cool as a cucumber.

My nurse listened, she didn't judge. She listened and said I wasn't crazy. She promised the doctor would call. I calmed down.

Next, God spoke to me, saying, "You are panicking because you think you've lost control over your body and you want it back. Remember the peace you felt a month ago, running the relay when you did not know about illness. You thought you had control then, but you didn't. Yet in your ignorance you experienced peace. Choose peace over control. It is attainable; control is not. Peace is not what is happening around you, it is what is happening inside you while circumstances swirl around you."

I would picture myself on a secure rock, focusing on the shore while the water cascaded around me, waiting for the tide to go out. After the water receded, I hopped off the rock and walked to shore, unharmed.

So I contended for my healing with peace as a weapon of war. I fought for it with sword and shield every day. When I got laughed at for believing Jesus healed me; when people got spooked just being around me because someone who is fighting for their life spooks people.

I remembered the account in the Bible when Jesus was asked to heal a girl who died before He could get to her. But He entered the ruler's house and saw the flute players and the noisy crowd. "Go away," He told them. "The girl is not dead, but asleep." And they laughed at Him. After the crowd had been put outside, Jesus went in and took the girl by the hand, and she got up, Matthew 9:24.

Cancer thrives and people die because we isolate those who are sick with it, not because of their immune system, but because we don't want to witness their struggle; it frightens us. But my battle was not to convince anyone else that I was well. It wasn't against the devil, because he was already defeated. My battle was to maintain my connection to Jesus and stand my ground in faith.

What I learned is that fear can be easier than faith. It can sometimes be easier to see a bad outcome and try to control it rather than release faith and hope for a good outcome because there's no more stress once you've accepted the negative outcome, it just is. My assignment was to make the effort to believe I was healed, to stand in faith and wait on the Lord, to declare my belief in a reality that hadn't happened yet and that I didn't control. For me, that was hard.

But in Luke 18:8, Jesus asks his disciples, "When the Son of Man comes, will he find faith on the earth?" My answer to this is YES, there will be faithful people on earth, we will be casting out demons, healing the sick, performing miracles, signs, and wonders as Christ did before He ascended. And, as He also said, "You will do greater works than these because I go to the Father." We cannot fail Him and so we must do the hard work of faith to help others and advance the kingdom.

I knew this was my assignment, so every day I declared that I would not die but live; to declare the works of the Lord. I would declare it after repeating John 10:18:

"No one takes it from me, but I lay it down of my own accord. I have authority to lay it down and authority to take it up again. This command I received from my Father." I declared that the command Jesus received from His Father was also a command for me, and I would never lay my life down for cancer.

I declare in the name of Jesus Christ of Nazareth whom I serve that I am not laying my life down for cancer; I'm not laying my life down for any sickness, disease, accident or infirmity. I am not laying my life down for another 60 years at least.

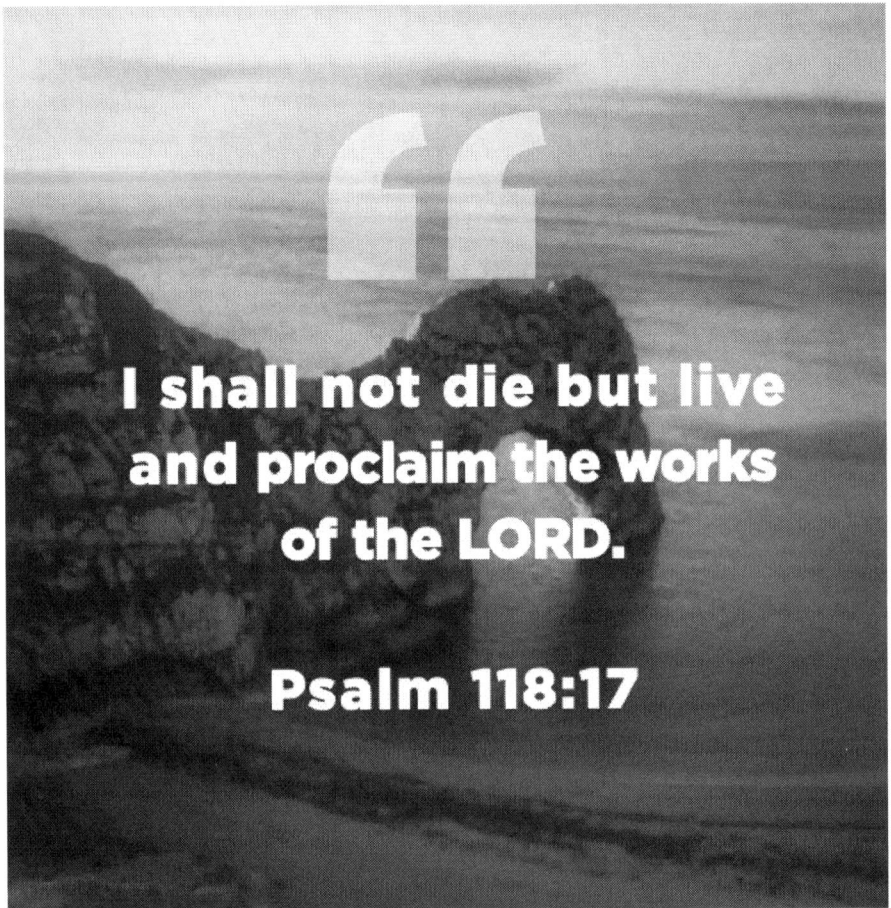

I shall not die but live and proclaim the works of the LORD.

Psalm 118:17

12

CHEMO #1

A Shot Across the Bow

Each chemo treatment has its own characteristics, largely dependent on their spot in the treatment cycle. Chemo #1 was like a warning shot across the bow. A display of power, meant to induce fear, with the sense of more to come. I got an end-to-end view of the toxicity cycle, then turned the corner on day seven, feeling better every day after that.

During those first six days, I felt like I was on Mars, a feeling that recurred the first two days of each treatment. I spent the time reflecting on my circumstances and what I learned. Over the prior two years, I had lost. Lost my retirement. Lost my position. Lost my family business and lost some family as part of that debacle. I lost my credit, my savings, my creativity and my free time. And then I lost my health.

I endured embarrassment, grief, humiliating days that just built on each other, my wall of shame and regret. I felt weighed down by my past and the five bags of chemicals I just had pumped into me, and as I struggled to remain positive the enemy spoke to me, telling me that my life insurance was the only way out; especially since I was sick, I was worth more to my family dead than alive.

During one of these moments, I heard the Holy Spirit ask me, "Which way are you going to go?" The question was randomly delivered while I sat at a red light, but I knew it was important, that my answer would establish my faith. It cemented my choices and illuminated the only way available for me, to walk through my darkness with belief. During this period, my mantra was stay, love, and fight for what I believed.

Belief—that space in your head that bridges who you are in Christ to who you are in the world. Christ knew His purpose, but even He had only belief to get Him through those moments of doubt on the cross when He needed His Father.

So I believed actively, I pursued belief daily. God surrounded me with elders and the Word. And I found that there was a side to belief I had never known before. A side that involved signs, wonders, miracles, the kinds of things I needed, really the only thing that could help. I learned that just because I had professed belief the day before didn't mean I wouldn't be shattered by circumstances the next day and have to regroup. I stopped being surprised that my wall of belief could take what I felt were air-to-surface homing missiles and stay standing, but I needed to rebuild a part of that wall every day.

When you are desperate, you will believe. God will take that effort on your part and make your belief into something glorious, but you have to believe dangerously, with everything you have, every thought, every spoken word, each moment must be dedicated to your belief.

And today, I can tell you this. I have never felt so loved and cared for by God, who ensured that during the process, my companions were Faith, Love and The Holy Spirit. Step by ordered step, I knew that He would lead me across the bridge, out of the darkness.

And He will do the same for you. Your gifts, your miracles, your healing waits for you, there is no difference between you and any other person God has healed.

Why then, would you deny yourself these gifts?

Picture your healing as a jar of golden light sitting on a table in a room, behind an unlocked door. You know it's there, and you are free to enter. Why would you walk past the door?

Take the doorknob in your hand, open that door, walk in and open the golden jar. It is yours, it is there for you and no one else.

If you're not ready to fully believe yet, then spend time reading about the miracles He's done for others. Here is a list that you can start with; read them and you will see for yourself what can happen.

- ❖ *Ridiculous Miracles*, Clarice Fluitt
- ❖ *Is That Really You, God?* Loren Cunningham
- ❖ *How to be Healed and Stay Healed*, Alice Cresswell
- ❖ *When Heaven Invades Earth; A Practical Guide to a Life of Miracles*, Bill Johnson
- ❖ *And Jesus Healed Them All*, Gloria Copeland
- ❖ *Healed of Cancer*, Dodie Olsteen
- ❖ *Diary of Miracles, Part I and II*, Alice Cresswell
- ❖ *Miracles from Heaven*, Christy Wilson Beam
- ❖ *A Touch from Heaven: A Little Boy's Story of Surgery, Heaven and Healing*, Neal Plyant

Yes, the enemy tried to tell me that suicide was a great choice. But love meant that I never considered that option. Instead, I took that as yet another attempt to steal something that would have to be paid back to me sevenfold. You can bet that if the enemy wants you gone, you have something incredible to contribute!

At the beginning of this book, I wrote that it is not a judgment call on those who fought cancer and died. After fighting cancer, I believe those who are in Christ and passed after fighting cancer are subject to a great reward in heaven. God keeps His promises and He promises beauty for ashes (Isaiah 61:3), He promises the restoration of the years the locusts have eaten (Joel 2:25), He promises that the thief must restore sevenfold everything that was stolen (Proverbs 6:31). Those whose faith choice was not made, or who made a choice not to believe in Christ, are still subject to God's mercy, and to healing through Jesus. When He walked the earth, Jesus healed all, and most of those he healed had no idea who he was.

Time is a construct for humans provided by God, and the reality of time is that everything is now. You can pray for those who have passed and God will hear your prayers. You can pray for the salvation of your atheist family member 10 years after they passed and God will hear your prayers. For God, a day is like a thousand years, and it only takes a moment for someone to accept His Son. That moment can happen at any "time." Never stop praying for that choice to be made.

In Exodus 33:19 God says, "I will have mercy on whom I will have mercy, and I will have compassion on whom I will have compassion." His will is the supreme decision; the highest hand that can be held in the game, the ultimate determination of the outcome. And He operates outside of time, He operates such that our final moments, even if we've spent our entire lives operating against Him, even if satan has persecuted us to the point of suicide, our final moments belong to Him. All power and mercy is wielded by Him, and He calls us, even then.

A haiku to my immune system after my first chemo infusion:
Please come back to me
My factory of healing
Much respect and love

13

THAT'S AMAZING!

I had my exam that happened prior to every chemo session, my first one since the diagnosis. The doctor did a quick breast exam. I watched his face change from mild concentration to a squinty-eyed focus. He stopped and took a step back, saying, "Do YOU feel anything in there?"

"Nope." But honestly, I never felt anything to begin with.

He stepped up again and went after my lump a second time, again stepping back, "It's gone. That's amazing, what a great response to your first treatment!"

I said, "I told you that between you and God, we would get this done!" He congratulated me and then said, "but you're going to finish your treatment, right?"

I told him that yes, I had committed to that and would do what he asked. He kept congratulating me, saying, "Good for you, good for you!"

Father, You walked me to this place of healing and I thank You so much for teaching me how to get here. I thank You for my healing Lord, thank you, thank you, thank you.

Then I declared that my treatments would do me no harm, they would not negatively affect my body or spirit. I also declared the ability to share with others how to do the same thing for themselves or those they love. In the name of Jesus Christ of Nazareth, whom I serve, Amen.

My daughter played basketball and I still took her to practice and games, wearing my beanie after my hair was gone and my germ mask depending on where I was in the chemo cycle. I accepted that not everybody was going to know what was going on with me so I had to be willing to be misunderstood when I pulled back from physical contact, or because I looked freaky in my wig and germ mask. But if you want to be a hero in your kid's life, you do what you have to do to show up. It only needed to make sense to her, anyway.

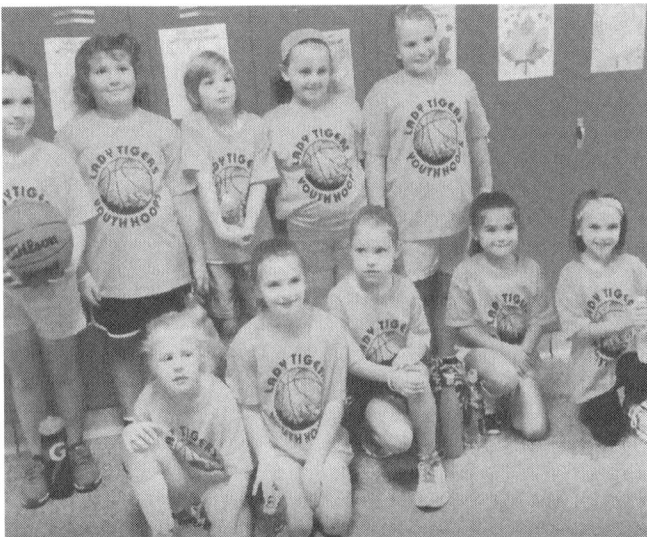

14

WEEK BEFORE CHEMO #2
A LITTLE PERSPECTIVE

I felt so normal right before chemo #2, almost 100%. But in one week, I knew I would be in the chemo DMZ. My nephew used to refer to the times when he and his unit in Afghanistan were behind enemy lines as "under the wire." Anything could happen, most of it bad, but necessary to complete the mission. I'm counting down seven days until I go under the wire again.

I still had my hair, but it was starting to give out. Single strands floated around me throughout the day and my wig sat on a stand staring at me like a dog that wanted to be walked. Until it happened, I couldn't imagine dropping all my hair, it was one more thing to add to the what-the-heck list. But life was about now, and at that point in the cycle, I was well, my hair was still there, and I felt better. There was no need to live anywhere else until I had to. The wire wasn't going anywhere; it would still be there.

Chemo #2 would happen right before Halloween.

It's impossible to overestimate the value of a sense of humor when dealing with stuff that life throws at you, but somehow cancer has managed to instill people with such fear we won't even laugh at it. But I come from sarcastic, macabre, train wreck comedian stock. So I played to my strengths with my Halloween costume and chose Gollum from The Lord of the Rings - nothing to buy!!!

There is very little comedy about cancer, which serves to keep it in some kind of sacrosanct space in people's heads. That kind of preciousness got to me and I searched for forms of expression that reduced the shrouded-in-mist veil of cancer to the juvenile, ADD cell expression-needing-a-time-out irritant that it was. I found some great videos that helped ease the tension and knock cancer down off the pedestal that we've put it on. One is a Ted Talk from Karen Mills, titled "Cancer is a Laughing Matter," and the other is a video from comic Jim Gaffigan, titled "Losing Arguments with your Wife after Her Brain Surgery."

15

HEALING AND PRAYER

The Women's Ministry at my church sent me encouragement. I considered them my elders of the church. James says in James 5:14:

Is any one of you sick? He should call the elders of the church to pray over him and anoint him with oil in the name of the Lord. I fulfilled this by reaching out to my elders before every chemo session to ask for prayer.

When I first asked others to pray for me, I knew the type of prayer I needed to receive—prayers that set in motion God's spiritual laws for healing. During his healing ministry, Jesus never asked if it was God's will for someone to be healed. The only time He ever asked God about His will was in the garden of Gethsemane regarding His sacrifice. It is always God's will to heal; always His will to restore. It is Jesus's will that we as heirs of salvation, heal as well as Him.

So instead of asking people to pray and hoping they didn't introduce doubt into my prayer life, I shared with them what I was praying for and asked them to stand in agreement with me. Once I started doing that, the prayers surrounding me were all positive, uplifting, and bold, prayers that made a demand on the covenant we have with God to manifest his promises in my life now.

16

CHEMO #2

CLIPPING THE MAST

Chemo #2 done, home, heading to Mars soon. My daughter acted out at school because it was an extreme homework night, and my husband stressed because of it. I was busy at work, but the reality remained: I COULD NOT TAP OUT. I resolved to needle-point this on a pillow. But then there was Mr. Rogers, my hero, who put everything in perspective, when he said, "There is no normal life that is free of pain. It's the very wrestling with our problems that can be the impetus for our growth."

I felt so much better this round, but day 3-5 is the toughest and was still to come. Still, I was thanking God and cleaning. My prayers were for no negative side effects from the chemo or the drugs to handle the side effects. I had the best care on the planet, and on Friday I would have my first exercise class at the hospital gym. I was looking forward to it.

I started my days saying "I walk in the favor of God" all day long, that amazing things happen for me, awesome things happen to me every day. And then I expected what I said to happen, and something always did.

Even when things happened that most would think were negative, I wasn't concerned because I knew what I believed and no weapon formed against me would prosper (Isaiah 54.17), everything the devil tried to steal from me—my peace, my families peace, businesses, income, the loose change in my car or the ultimate, my life—everything was tracked and he must restore sevenfold what he stole from me. And I would never give up demanding recompense. Never. Ever.

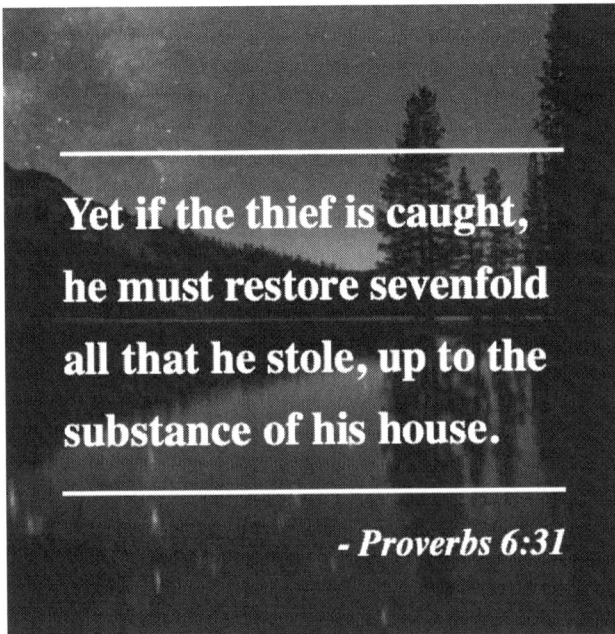

Yet if the thief is caught, he must restore sevenfold all that he stole, up to the substance of his house.

- Proverbs 6:31

Chemo Session #2, Day 3

I felt covered by God for healing. I was sluggish with break-through joint and body pain. The toxins seemed to focus on exiting my body through my skin and joints. Over the next two days I sort of tracked them moving around inside of me then exiting. I focused on love in my body, on being covered by Jesus, and soldiering through it with prayer. I "ran across" prayers, memes, and blog posts that seemed to be meant directly for me. I continued to find support from other believers, and since I spent most of my time online, I found believers there like Sandi Krakowski, who said, in essence, hang in there, body, Sunday is coming.

#Jesusthankyouformyhealing

Sandi Krakowski November 2, 2016 ·

Are you in physical pain? Struggling with disease? As you believe for healing and do all you can to support your body PROPHESY over yourself. I love you body! You're beautiful! You've carried me through pain and trauma and I love you. You are strong, healing, coming into alignment with heaven and I love you!" Don't be angry at your body. Our subconscious mind responds to what we say and think. LOVE yourself, all of you. Your body has carried you through all of life! ♥☐

Sandi Krakowski
November 2, 2016 · 🌐

When God builds something it's always ironic the opposition AND the support that comes. We can focus on the attacks OR we can focus on the angels working behind the scenes. Some threats are like a big black bear with no teeth! All bark- no bite. That's the PROPHETIC WORD of this hour. All bark- no bite. No one can stop what God is building. No demon, no human. Stay faithful! #GodsGotYourBack #IDeclareVictory

CHEMO SESSION #2, DAY 5

Last zombie day, then I start moving forward again. Still, when I'm asked by family what it's like having cancer, chemo, "what's been most difficult for you?" I am unable, quite literally unable, to speak anything but praise, thankfulness and gratitude. I believe the Holy Spirit has placed a guard on my tongue about what I say relative to this experience. My faith, wellness, healing, depends on my ability to see beyond what is and call my experiences good, to view my situation from a vantage point of opportunity bestowed, blessings received, and victory secured from a place of real danger.

So I share some specifics about the route the drugs take through my system, the daily progression I feel as the toxins go after my stir-crazy cells; but I'm always quick to add that the cancer is gone, I know that. I'm healed, and I'm well, I am to give no attention to the illness itself, only to the miracles surrounding it in my life.

This round of chemo, I had to add that we Americans crave the most ridiculous foods. After my second infusion, I was unable to watch television commercials, with their zoomed in pictures of hamburgers melting with grease, cheese and piled with fried onions, or the layered, sugar-upon-sugar deserts we devour, some with inch-and-a-half towers of frosting or solid candy exteriors, drizzled with even more icing. Even today, two years later, I have to look away and hold my stomach at the sight of over processed piles of grease and sugar we call food. We have made it illegal to sell tobacco and alcohol to people without meeting age requirements, but we will whole-heartedly support promoting foods that are just as deadly to us as tobacco and alcohol, with no disclaimers at all. I'm thankful for the "food filter" that chemotherapy still provides me; nausea is a symptom that returns immediately upon seeing this type of food today and makes it a no brainer to turn it down.

I was blessed to run across this beautiful blessing from Theresa Dedmon:

I would love to just speak to everyone out there just to tune out anything else that you're doing and begin to ask Holy Spirit what he loves about you and how he's created you to be. And I want you to forget about any other voice in your life and look at how God has created you.

And right now I bless the way that God looks at you right now, how he's created you to be. I bless the dreams that you have and I say, Father, activate them in creative ways beyond what they could ever imagine. Release the blocks. Release the things that they're going to be doing.

Lord, as they start to partner with you, I pray that there would be a release from everything that has limited them to think that their life is ordinary and I pray that it would be transformational and there would be a supernatural grace to now take a risk, start to open up your heart and give away what you've been given from God.
Theresa Dedmon

17
HEALING VISION BOARD

I was feeling creative. So many showed me kindness through cards, words, and memes, that it gave me an idea. I created a healing vision board on the wall in my office. I assembled pictures, made more pictures, and cleared the space for it. I considered myself to be co-creating with God; it felt like riding a wave, and I drew strength and encouragement from it.

I included pictures of my ancestors. They had something to do with my healing, too. I have always known that they prayed for me, literally over a hundred years ago, for my salvation and my future. Others have known trauma, challenge, and illness, but their story is part of mine, too. When I looked closely at their faces, I saw strength, support and encouragement. It's as if they were looking straight at me and saying, "Well? What are you waiting for?"

WHEN SOMEONE OFFERS TO HELP SAY YES
DON'T WORRY ABOUT MAC N' CHEESE
CIRCLE THE WAGONS AND DO WHAT YOU NEED TO DO TO HELP
YOURSELF
KISSES FROM KIDS ALWAYS HELP
MY FAVORITE BOOK WAS (IS) LOVE, MEDICINE, AND MIRACLES
BY BERNIE SIEGEL
BUT YOU WILL FIND WHAT RESONATES WITH YOU
AND EVERYONE AND EVERYTHING EXCEPT THESE FEW CELLS WANT
YOU TO BE WELL
IT'S A TIDAL WAVE AGAINST THOSE STUPID CELLS
YOU'VE GOT THIS - PAM JANSON

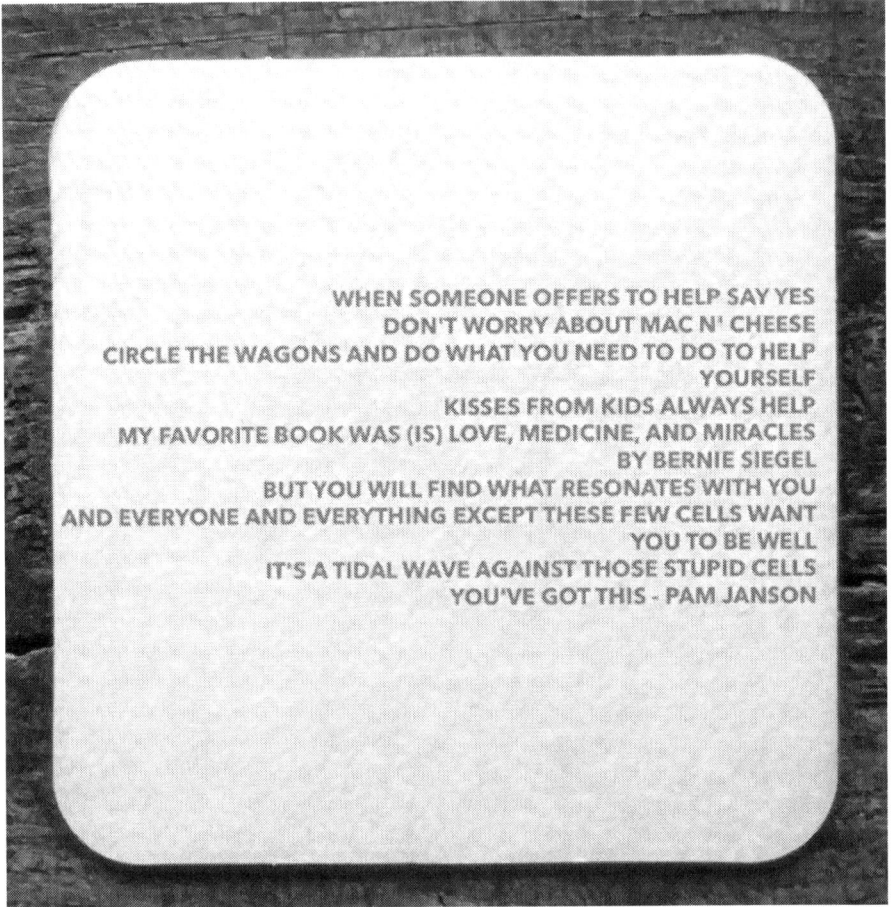

I framed every encouragement I received and hung them, creating a giant healing vision board on the wall, and then I videotaped the wall and sent it to everyone who contributed to it. Father, thank You for this project! Guide me so that it glorifies You. In Jesus's name, Amen.

As I rolled through chemo #2, I felt an urging and a burden regarding healing as an everyday occurrence for all of us, especially for those in the body of Christ.

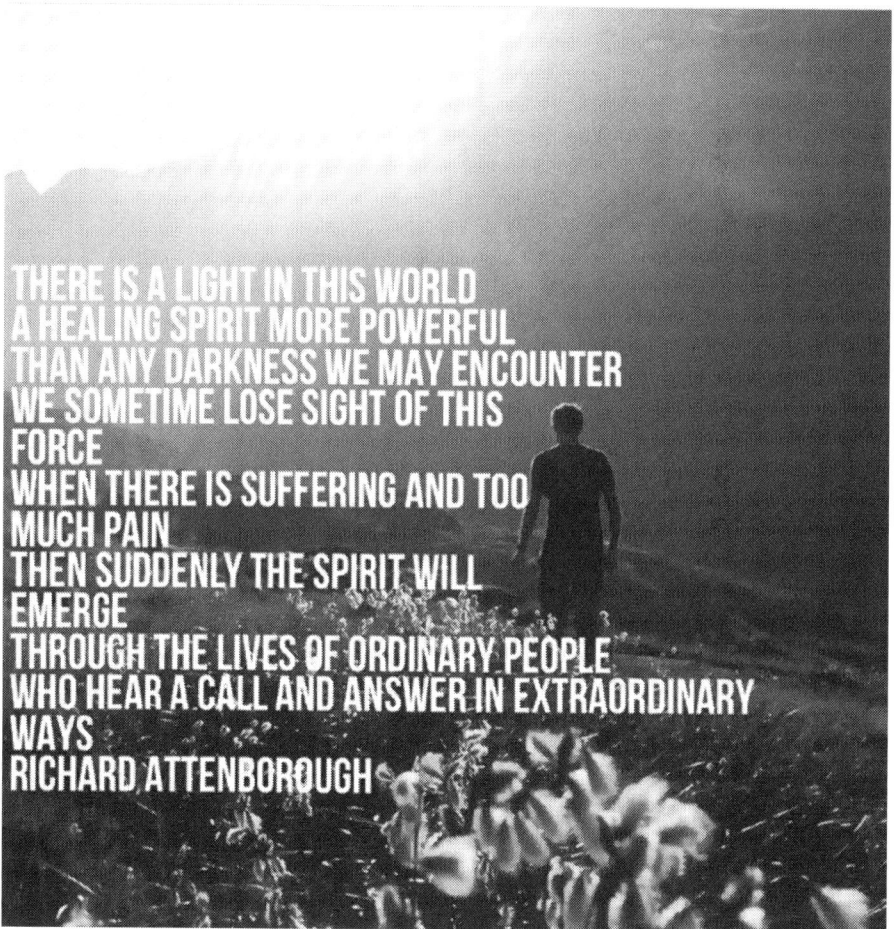

THERE IS A LIGHT IN THIS WORLD
A HEALING SPIRIT MORE POWERFUL
THAN ANY DARKNESS WE MAY ENCOUNTER
WE SOMETIME LOSE SIGHT OF THIS
FORCE
WHEN THERE IS SUFFERING AND TOO
MUCH PAIN
THEN SUDDENLY THE SPIRIT WILL
EMERGE
THROUGH THE LIVES OF ORDINARY PEOPLE
WHO HEAR A CALL AND ANSWER IN EXTRAORDINARY
WAYS
RICHARD ATTENBOROUGH

Isaiah 53 says, "But he was wounded for our transgressions, he was bruised for our iniquities: the chastisement of our peace was upon him, and with his stripes we are healed."

To me, this meant that Jesus took cancer on the cross and it died with Him. The spiritual burden I felt was to illuminate this fact and make it specific to cancer; i.e., we need to take our God-given authority over cancer and manhandle it out of existence. I prayed and asked Jesus to please show me how. I was learning every day by visiting mystics, healers, gathering healing prayers and not giving up, like Jacob wrestling with the angel, or the woman in Luke who wore out the king with her constant request for recompense, and Caleb requesting his portion of land to fight for, because at 80 years old, he declared himself fully able to fight and win. I declared over and over that I would not give up, and that any different outcome meant something was stolen from me, and that something would have to be restored sevenfold. I kept a tally board of everything the devil had stolen from me and I added to it every day. I was not letting him off the hook for a single thing. My peace, my family's peace, time with my family and friends, medical bills, lost business, my hair, breasts, sleep, white blood cells, I got specific!

I reminded the devil when God looks at me, He sees me through His son—whole and healthy—that in Psalm 91 God promised me long life, honor and His salvation, and I wasn't laying down my life for another 60 years at least. That I would watch my daughter grow up and help care for my grandchildren.

That my husband and I would work for as long as we wanted and enjoy retirement for even longer. I didn't say these things in a taunting way, I said them in the authority of Jesus Christ. I spoke out my future no matter what I was being told about my present.

Satan may be trying to take something from you, but it's important that you know it was never his to take, and that in God's kingdom, that means he owes you. And you can hold him to that sevenfold recompense after Proverbs 6:31. We have been given the power to hold him accountable and should do so.

I also spent time considering Genesis 50:20: You intended to harm me, but God intended it for good, to accomplish what is now being done, the saving of many lives.

I made scripture art for this verse so I could meditate on it and imagine all the ways that lives could be saved as a result of this attempt to harm me. That is ultimately how this book began to take shape and why I have confidence that this book will reach the hands of people who need it; because God says that His Word will accomplish what He said it would. In Isaiah 55:11, He says, "so is my word that goes out from my mouth: It will not return to me empty but will accomplish what I desire and achieve the purpose for which I sent it."

> ## You intended to harm me, but God intended it for good to accomplish what is now being done, the saving of many lives.
>
> ### - Genesis 50:20

The effects of chemo sessions were building on each other and the cumulative effect was that it took longer for me to hit the turnaround day. I finally got there on day ten. I started to fear because I felt weak, but God sent His Word, reminding me of my first lesson:

"Only do not rebel against the LORD; and do not fear the people of the land, for they will be our prey. Their protection has been removed from them, and the LORD is with us; do not fear them." Numbers 14:9

It was more than behavior coaching; it was saying they are the prey, their protection has been removed from them. The implication was more than safety. It was also about advancing with the confidence of the Lord backing me.

Once again the Holy Spirit reminded me that to fear is to be disobedient. In effect, clipping my mast if I let it happen. It worked like a Jedi mind trick. I practiced this approach repeatedly, every time I felt a wave of fear, panic, anxiety, begin to wash over me. I would stop the wave the moment I felt it gathering and heard God's voice say DO NOT FEAR; REMEMBER YOUR TRAINING. Then I would pray aloud:

And now, we break the assignment of the enemy to continuously afflict me with loss and fear. And I declare in the name of Jesus Christ of Nazareth whom I serve, that all trauma, all lack of any kind, all illness, infirmity, accident, injury or attack LEAVES NOW. And Jesus Himself restores what has been stolen from me. Jesus is the God of restoration, and He always restores to a place that is greater than before, therefor I now possess greater health, greater spiritual growth, greater abundance, greater security. Thank you for my restoration Lord. Thank you for my healing.

I would follow it with spoken scripture that prophesied my healing:

I have given you authority to trample on snakes and scorpions and to overcome all the power of the enemy; nothing will harm you. Luke 10:19

Fear is an illusion the enemy uses to execute his purpose; it is the reason he is called the father of lies. But I had been practicing this for a few weeks and didn't think it would continue to be a problem; however, I needed to renew an all-out campaign against fear, reminding myself over and over that, outside the realm of actual danger, fear is smoke and mirrors. False Evidence Appearing Real.

We make the enemy's job easier when we give fear a foothold, like allowing frightening, awful information into our minds through what we watch, read and hear. I stopped watching crime shows and horror movies and when my family watched films that contained violence, I closed my eyes during the scenes and said that I would not allow Satan to get a foothold through whatever was on the screen.

When I adopted my daughter, the agency we worked with talked about ways to bond during our first year together and how important those first 12 months would be. She would sit in my lap and we would find videos on the internet about soldiers coming home to surprise their families, people finding lost dogs, and other videos where families found each other and were joyful. We shared those emotional moments and it helped us bond and grow together as a family.

Thinking back to those times, I chose to fill my mind with what my body needed. I ran internet searches on words like healing, joy, winning, and then viewed the images associated with those words. Then I searched for videos with the same or similar words and watched them. I strongly encourage you to try this, especially if you are battling illness. Watch and listen, even if you are multi-tasking, that's fine; just keep the positive inputs coming as often as you can.

I also used imagery to support me. Here is an amazing guided imagery practice that blessed me. Search for a video of Secretariat's record-breaking 3rd win in the Triple Crown, at Belmont Stakes.

While you are watching this magnificent creature run (I've owned horses and do not condone racing these animals; however, Secretariat was a horse that knew his purpose, and running was his THING), repeat with the announcer his comments below using your name instead of Secretariat, and using the illness that you have overcome:

Valerie is in a good position!

Valerie has taken the lead! The lead is increasing!

Valerie is moving like a tremendous machine!

Valerie is in the home stretch!

Valerie has opened a huge lead from cancer!

AMAZING - UNBELIEVABLE PERFORMANCE!

VALERIE IS THE WINNER!!! VALERIE BEATS CANCER!!!

DAY 10 AFTER CHEMO #2

Feeling better, no appetite, but I'm getting calories and will look forward to enjoying food again a year from now.

I'm heading into cold weather, the holidays, all good prospects unless you are someone who has to limit their exposure to people and germs; then it becomes about the most challenging time of the year. I've started speaking life over my body and my immune system and death over any germs, illness or infirmity.

18

REPENT, FORGIVE, HEAL

In Acts 3, Peter heals a lame man and then addresses the crowd about healing. After healing him, Peter explains the covenant blessing to the crowd, "And you are heirs of the prophets and of the covenant God made with your fathers. He said to Abraham, 'Through your offspring all peoples on earth will be blessed.' When God raised up his servant, he sent him first to you to bless you by turning each of you from your wicked ways."

This covenant blessing belongs to all who follow Christ. This blessing allows you to receive healing and to take up the mantle of rights and responsibilities of a believer. Peter went on to say:

Repent, then, and turn to God, so that your sins may be wiped out, that times of refreshing may come from the Lord, and that he may send the Messiah, who has been appointed for you—even Jesus.

While the man held on to Peter and John, all the people were astonished and came running to them in the place called Solomon's Colonnade. When Peter saw this, he said to them: "Fellow Israelites, why does this surprise you? Why do you stare at us as if by our own power or godliness we had made this man walk? The

God of Abraham, Isaac and Jacob, the God of our fathers, has glorified his servant Jesus. You handed him over to be killed, and you disowned him before Pilate, though he had decided to let him go. You disowned the Holy and Righteous One and asked that a murderer be released to you. You killed the author of life, but God raised him from the dead. We are witnesses of this. By faith in the name of Jesus, this man whom you see and know was made strong. It is Jesus's name and the faith that comes through him that has completely healed him, as you can all see.

"Now, fellow Israelites, I know that you acted in ignorance, as did your leaders. But this is how God fulfilled what he had foretold through all the prophets, saying that his Messiah would suffer. Repent, then, and turn to God, so that your sins may be wiped out, that times of refreshing may come from the Lord, and that he may send the Messiah, who has been appointed for you— even Jesus. Heaven must receive him until the time comes for God to restore everything, as he promised long ago through his holy prophets. For Moses said, 'The Lord your God will raise up for you a prophet like me from among your own people; you must listen to everything he tells you. Anyone who does not listen to him will be completely cut off from their people.'

"Indeed, beginning with Samuel, all the prophets who have spoken have foretold these days. And you are heirs of the prophets and of the covenant God made with your fathers. He said to Abraham, 'Through your offspring all peoples on earth will be blessed.' When God raised up his servant, he sent him first to you to bless you by turning each of you from your wicked ways." Acts 3:11-26

I sat at my kitchen table, which had become my prayer corner, my warrior room, and sobbed uncontrollably, the words from Acts 3 reaching me with effortless conviction. At first, I imagined I was crying because…who wouldn't? My situation was grave and I had a young family to protect. But when I went deeper, I knew that my hardened heart compounded my situation. Unforgiveness, bitterness, judgment and frustration that gave way to a fortress of anger in my mind. These emotional strongholds were capable of weakening my immune system and holding back my healing and the Holy Spirit knew it, knew I needed to repent not only for my past willingness to allow them but also the tendency to turn to these responses when tempted. When the alternative is death, even the most painful injuries at the hands of another person seem petty. And forgiving others gave way to forgiving myself for my own mistakes. I cried to my Abba Daddy for forgiveness for all the foolish choices I had made in my life, every person I hurt, every opportunity I squandered and every time I took my holiness, the light I carried within me, for granted, grieving the Holy Spirit and limiting my potential.

At that time, I would start each day with my devotions and during my readings, eventually give way to heartbreaking tears as I wept over my past behavior, times I had hurt others, times I had been hurt. Then, when it was time to wake my daughter and tend to school, my job and family, the tears would turn off until the next morning. This went on for over a week until there were no more tears left and the raw pain of my shortcomings and hurtful memories no longer carried the edge they once had.

I felt that my repentance was accepted, I was humbled again and again, and my heart felt new, with more room for compassion and more tools for how to manage situations that tested my personal, professional and emotional limits. Chief among them was to value and protect my holiness and to pursue peace in my daily living; two concepts that guide me today.

To protect my holiness required a commitment to two things: to limit my exposure to the unholy and to partake in the holy. It was that simple. And again, the Holy Spirit gifted me with an interest in the holy, through reading, watching and participating in pastimes that focused on things that were positive, loving and inspiring while my appetite for the unholy was as nauseous as food during chemo. My language, choice of music, movies, and books began to change, to evolve to the positive, and these choices made me happier, more resilient, less selfish and self-focused.

For example, I was so impressed with the medical teams that helped me that I would take gifts for them when I arrived for infusions. "Gifting" others became an opportunity I genuinely looked forward to. Expressing gratitude to and for others, with things as small as a jar of candy or a set of angel wings for their desk gave me joy, and it was truly surprising how rarely they received things like this. Here was a whole team of people whose jobs are to care for some of the sickest humans on the planet and they were rarely thanked for their work. For the record, they were handling extremely toxic chemicals on the daily as well. I didn't want to fall into the trap of being so wrapped up in the illness that I couldn't see the sacrifices others were making for me.

And they were so surprised and grateful to be noticed, but it was me who reaped the benefits of choosing to express my sincere appreciation for them. By doing so, I strengthened the shield of love around me, the healing light of love in my heart burned brighter. Giving, even during times when I was in a chemo fog, became an antidote for me.

I would walk around the infusion center after receiving treatment and talk to some of the other patients, praying with them if they wanted to. I met people who were there receiving their 20th, their 30th infusion. Words cannot express the quiet bravery of these individuals, many there alone, yet some were smiling, asking me about my situation, encouraging me, telling me what to expect next, assuring me that I would be fine. I smiled back, agreed with them, and told them how much their words meant to me. There are soldiers, true soldiers of God, serving in infusion centers everywhere, providing encouragement, bearing each other's burdens, even as they bear their own.

I chose to view my infusions as times of special care; I called it my day spa. I would rest in a heated recliner with a warm blanket and work on my laptop while I ate my "last meal" before heading to Mars and a couple of weeks of non-stop nausea. Infusions usually lasted a few hours, so I could take conference calls and complete my work in peace.

I started praying loaves and fishes over the hair on my head. As in, "like the loaves and fishes, my hair will grow again in abundance!" I repeated every time I threw away a hair blob. And there was always more. I donated the first 8 inches of hair and declared it as seed sown. It occurred to me that, if I was going to lose some of my hair, the addition of false eyelashes could counteract the loss and make me look less alien/zombie-like. My good friend applied them expertly and I was excited to see the improvement. Unfortunately, my new look was now Alien/Zombie-Goes-To-Vegas, primarily because my eyebrows were almost gone. But the lashes were glued on, so my family and I had to deal with it for the rest of my treatments.

Chemo #3 was the next day, and I was feeling normal, as I did when I was in my third week of the cycle. Our family came to my home for Thanksgiving and we had so much to be thankful for! We had dinner that night so I could cook and eat with everyone. I had already had the flu and a killer cold, but my immune system held up, and my numbers were good, praise God. I needed my blood cell counts to be decent so I could knock out the third chemo and be halfway home.

I visited the Rhoda Wise Miracle House in Canton, Ohio. I went there every chemo to pray and petition for healing. She has an amazing story, and I found her by "accident."

I used to watch Mother Angelica, a vibrant, warm, amazing nun on TV. When I was first diagnosed, I surfed the web for healing videos and remembered her. When I Googled Mother Angelica Healing, up came Rhoda Wise and Miracle House. It turned out that Mother Angelica was originally from Canton, Ohio and as a young woman, she had a serious stomach ailment, so her mother took her to see Rhoda Wise at her home (now Miracle House) in Canton, where she was cured. Today, Rhoda is in the final stages of canonization in the Catholic Church, and her home was only 25 minutes away! This is what I mean when I say that God has miracles for you every single day.

During my lunch hour, I drove to her home, toured Miracle House, and shared my situation with the team at her home while they prayed over me. I felt peace when I was there and a deeper connection to the saints in the Catholic Church who suffered for Jesus. I considered her another elder of the church that I went to for healing. Rhoda Wise had a very personal, real relationship with Jesus that resulted in many miracles for her and others. I was grateful that, once again, I was given the chance to learn about someone who sacrificed for others. I gathered holy water from her home and took it with me every time I had chemotherapy and it comforted me because it made me feel closer to the miraculous world that Jesus inhabits.

Rhoda was a healer, a stigmatist and a mentor, but everything she did came from her relationship with Jesus. She suffered physically and mentally during her life, yet her goal became to suffer on purpose. She prayed for people, for souls and for entire nations. Her life became one of purposeful prayer and mystical suffering. While I was in her home, I could feel the presence of Christ as I walked from room to room and listened to her story.

I converted to Catholicism as an adult largely because they would have me. While walking into Christ the King Church at the age of 26 to learn about the conversion process, I plopped my gum in the holy water, thinking it was some kind of wastebasket on the wall. After hearing the sound of my gum dropping into water, I fished it out, looking over my shoulder like a thief, mortified by my ignorance. That was the beginning of my relationship with

Jesus and the Catholic church. Me making mistakes and them spiritually rolling their eyes and forgiving me. Me wondering what I was doing and how I could possibly be a worthwhile recruit for the kingdom and them, patiently waiting until I got myself together.

To me, the Catholic church was home and I still feel welcome anywhere in the world. During my treatments and any other times of crisis in my life, regardless my current church membership, catholic mass remains the place where I feel welcome, touched, forgiven, and blessed to move forward, so the discovery of Rhoda Wise and the role she played in healing was a gift to me.

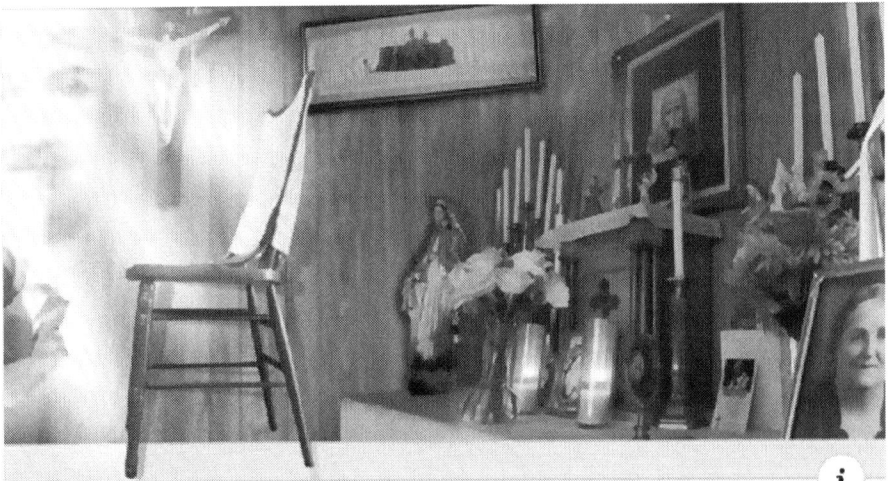

WWW.RHODAWISE.COM
Rhoda Wise | The Official Rhoda Wise Website – Miracle House
"Cures more wonderful than your own will take place on this spot."...

19

Chemo #3 – Torpedo to the Stern

Day 2 after chemo #3. Thanksgiving was easy breezy. My family held Thanksgiving dinner a day early so I could participate and taste the food. We had a party at the house, another no-no, but I did not pick up anything from the crowd and we had a wonderful time.

God was leading me somewhere and it gave me hope. I would pray daily: Father I am in alignment with You, take me where you want me to be! I declare in the name of Jesus Christ of Nazareth whom I serve that I Am WITH YOU! Amen.

I'm reading *Divine Healing Made Simple* by the Praying Medic, an EMT in Tacoma Washington who has had a healing ministry for years. He gave very practical advice on how to heal others and shared many miraculous healings that the Holy Spirit worked through him. The way he explains it is:

Healing is warfare, but it's warfare done from a place of rest. Our victory comes from what Jesus has already done; all we do is inform the world that the victory has been won. Once you begin to heal the sick, the enemy is likely to take notice and bring some resistance your way. Don't be afraid; it's only a fear campaign to get you to quit. Rest in the knowledge that you are more than a conqueror (see Rom. 8: 37).

THE PRAYING MEDIC

The phrase, warfare done from a place of rest, stood out to me. This was how the Holy Spirit drew my attention to areas I needed to study. Warfare done from a place of rest. I noticed during the healing videos I watched that the people I saw who healed others—Alice Cresswell, Gloria Copeland, Bill Johnson, the Praying Medic—did not use animated language or elaborate prayers. There was no yelling, arm waving or finger-pointing, only questions and prayers. But the questions and prayers carried with them a tone of authority, a knowingness that imparted a sense that they were on the same page with God and understood what needed to happen to heal.

And they all said that there were times when healing didn't happen; but when that occurred, they didn't raise their voice or denounce the sick person as evil. Jesus healed all is what the Bible says, but His disciples could not. They brought to Him a man so beset by demons that they could not heal Him, only Jesus could. When the disciples asked why they failed to heal, Jesus told them, in Mark 9:29, "This kind can come out only by prayer." The King James Version says, "This kind can come forth only by prayer and fasting." But when Matthew relates the same situation, he shares more of Jesus's comments. In Matthew 17:19-21, it says: Then the disciples came to Jesus in private and asked, "Why couldn't we drive it out?" He replied, "Because you have so little faith. Truly I tell you, if you have faith as small as a mustard seed, you can say to this mountain, 'Move from here to there,' and it will move. Nothing will be impossible for you."

So clearly there was some element to faith that enabled healing but that wasn't as accessible as simply saying what I wanted to happen out loud or speaking scripture over someone. I wanted something foolproof. It seemed like the only solution had to be some type of procedure, skill or anointing that guaranteed healing, but the more I read, watched and participated in healing moments, the less I saw that fell into the category of This Will Work Every Time. It was just the opposite; all kinds of people could heal all kinds of illness, accidents, and injuries, but each one had a story of when it hadn't happened, and we all know of people, many of whom we love, whose healing didn't happen.

I asked the Holy Spirit about this and kept reading about more people who healed. Their results were often successful, not always, but often, and many in ways I had never thought of. Limbs were restored, bodily organs were renewed, stage four cancer was dissolved away. And not all healings happened as a result of instant, miracle cures, either. Fields of study exist around cancer that focus on cures as a result of non-typical medical protocols, many with great success. I found the same to be true for heart disease, diabetes, and obesity.

The more I looked, the greater the variety of healing options I found, along with direct proof that these options worked for some people, sometimes. And many of the practitioners were not Christian; they were not operating out of a place of personal testimony, yet they healed Christians and others. They were God's instrument in the healing of Christians, though, which, to the sick person, was just as valuable.

I realized two things as a result of researching healing: That the common thread through this web of outcomes was not the outcome itself, it was the process of being led to an outcome, which was unique to the individual. To me, this was evidence of the Holy Spirit operating in our lives to "work all things together for our good" Romans 8:28. Our sovereign God, accessible by the work of His Son, Jesus, operating through the Holy Spirit, propels us, informs us, positions us, directs us, executes whatever is necessary to get us where we need to be to heal.

I also found that the key to someone's ability to heal was the same for a medical doctor as it was for a spiritual healer. The common denominator was not the perfect prayer or procedure, it was *practice*. By far the accounts of those who healed spiritually all started with an inability to heal, but they were willing to continue to try; to embarrass themselves to heal, honestly.

That was the situation the Praying Medic was referring to when he said, "Once you begin to heal the sick, the enemy is likely to take notice and bring some resistance your way." Resistance often took the form of flat out failure, over and over again. I learned firsthand how effective the failure to heal can be as I did a mental check down on everything involved in that failure. Primarily being a loss of faith on the part of the person who needed to be healed, not to mention the personal cost of attempting something in public, in the name of Jesus, that Just. Didn't. Work.

So my assignment became to start healing—stranger, acquaintance, family member or friend, anyone I could work with along with the Holy Spirit.

I was nervous but I felt ready and God allowed me to pray for a newborn little boy. He was 3 weeks old with RSV and had been put in Neonatal ICU. I asked the Holy Spirit if this was where He wanted me to pray, from a distance like this, and the response was yes.

I declared in the name of Jesus Christ of Nazareth, whom I serve, that little James's RSV was gone from that moment, that all illness, infirmity, accident, injury and demonic forces would leave him and his body at that moment and not return. And that Jesus himself would restore James; that Jesus always restores to a place greater than before, so James would experience greater health, greater protection, love, and security; all in the name of Jesus, Amen. I prayed this each day and would check for updates.

Within a week, James was fine, eating well, and home from the hospital. I realize that this was not the same experience as healing a person with an instant result, but it was a start, and I was encouraged.

I began asking people who were fighting cancer with me, my Day Spa mates, if I could pray for them. We knew where we each were in the battle, and cancer patients tend to be very medically oriented. We are erudite when it comes to the illness. I found that I could develop prayers for them that brought them peace before surgery, or strengthen them before their next infusion, which is critical when blood counts impact their ability to receive chemo.

I decided that healing is a combination of practice and practitioner; that there are people, places, and teams that heal; and these healers are good at it because they heal often, they practice healing in the same way that physicians practice their area of specialization. Finding them is a coordinated effort in the miraculous that the Holy Spirit will orchestrate for you. Ask Him; He will guide you in a way personal to you, and you will have your own healing story. Or read some of the authors I've listed in this book and, as Alice Cresswell says, "Give it a go!"

I list many of the healers and healing teams I have come into contact with throughout the book, but there are more. There are as many healers as there are people who need to be healed. The Holy Spirit operates through people, and there are billions of us.

As I read about healing, names would come up of people and teams whose abilities were really strong. I would check their web pages and see if they were ever physically close to my location. If they were, I went to them. I've already mentioned that a woman,

Rhoda Wise, currently in the canonization process for her healing miracles, among other miracles, had lived her life only 25 minutes away from me. The internet brought many of these individuals within reach as well. My only caution is that none of the healing events that I attended required money from me. Please don't be duped by people who attach money to healing. Jesus said to His disciples as He charged them with the responsibility along with the ability to heal, "freely you have received, freely give" Matthew 10:8. This doesn't mean that a donation wouldn't be accepted; however, it is not a requirement in any way and none of the people and teams who prayed for me ever even discussed money. Never. Ever.

As I reached out to pray for others, as I asked strangers who were sick, or limping, if I could pray for them, I began to feel that certainty inside, a solidness in my thinking that established itself as a place of rest. I was no longer hoping I could heal; instead, I knew that in some way and to some extent, what I was doing *was healing*. The outcome was something I had no control over, but the desire to heal and the tools to promote it, those I had and I used them every day. The desire to heal others became a daily practice for me. Today, part of my devotions is focused on praying for the healing of others. Every single day. And I am never at a loss when it comes to someone to pray for. The Holy Spirit brings a person or situation to mind easily. Praying for the healing of someone has become a habit. On social media, or the news, whenever it is evident that healing is needed, which is daily, often hourly, I am honored to assist through prayer. By praying for the healing of others, I built my faith and also participated in one of God's greatest mysteries, that what you give for others, you receive for yourself. I am convinced that part of my healing was as a result of praying healing over others, and that staying healed involves continually giving away healing prayer over others.

CHEMO #3, DAY 4

I was not feeling well. It was the toughest round so far, and I couldn't keep food down. I began a practice of leaving the dinner table early, "to start cleaning up." I would take my plate of gravel, because that's what any type of food turned to in my mouth once I took a bite, and head to the kitchen, where I would talk with my family from a distance. This way I could manage nausea but still be with them during dinnertime.

Despite my state, I had an amazing morning filled with God's grace.

I keep up with Sid Roth and his show, "It's Supernatural," and one day, there was a woman on named Joan Gieson, who said she had worked with Kathryn Kuhlman and had a healing ministry out of St. Louis. Joan is a servant of Christ who has worked in healing ministries for decades, and

I found an out-of-print copy of her book, *Things Thought Impossible*, and learned of all the miraculous works God did through her for the people of her community for food, shelter, Christmas dinners and healings. She inspired me because of her unrelenting faith, hope, and belief in what God is capable of doing. Through Christ, she healed her daughter of grave illness, along with others throughout her lifetime.

On this morning, I noticed that there was a phone number in the back of her book and decided I would call that number and see if there was a healing service she was attending anywhere near me in 2017. I also wanted to know how I could send a prayer request for my daughter. I called the number and a woman answered. I told her that I had seen Joan Gieson on Sid Roth's show and got her book and what a blessing it was to me, and we just started talking. She prayed over my daughter, blessing her, covering her, contending for her, and then I told her about my health situation.

She was very compassionate and brought up things about me that she could not have known, like how I spend my time in prayer, what times of day, what my daughter and I have been through together. I knew I was getting a word of knowledge as well as healing declarations over both my daughter and me.

At the end of the conversation, I thanked her again, and she asked for my phone number so she could call me. Then she told me that it was Joan Gieson herself that I was speaking with the whole time. I began to cry and told her how much her book had helped me and that I was amazed that she had picked up the phone when I called! She told me she was honored to pray for my daughter and me and that we would talk again soon.

One of the things she mentioned in her book when she discussed her daughter's illness was, "If you need a mighty miracle, you must go where God's presence is." This reminded me again of how important it is to get in the presence of God. God was present throughout our whole conversation; He was the one who orchestrated it! I declared my thankfulness and gratitude for the miracle of introducing me to Joan Gieson, first in a television show, then in a book, then on a phone call in real life! Father God, Jesus, Holy Spirit, thank you for this beautiful miracle, thank You for making me feel so loved today; thank you for my healing. In Jesus's mighty name, Amen!

DAYS 5-10 OF CHEMO #3

I was unable to get off the couch. What I didn't realize was that I was not taking my side effect protocol correctly and I had shorted myself a whole dose before the infusion. Between the meds protocol mistake and the accumulated effects of my third chemo, it took me twelve days, five of them spent more or less on the couch, to hit the turn around.

For people who went through chemo years ago, decades ago, before there was a decent side effect protocol, I salute you, admire you, and stand in awe. Words struggle to express the triage of nausea, weakness, and distress that multiple bodily systems experience. My entire body was a heaving pile of chaotic hot mess; as if something, a key component of bodily peace and order, was missing. Overlay that with steroid-induced emotional overreaction and you are a malnourished, abandoned infant in an adult body.

I cried to the Lord in my distress and He heard me. I was still a malnourished hot mess, but not abandoned, never alone, never without Him. I declared healing over myself and sought prayer from others. I let others help me because I had to, and I learned that they had been trying to help me all along. My brokenness was His opportunity to pour love into my life. I still cried often, but my tears were about finally seeing and accepting love in my life.

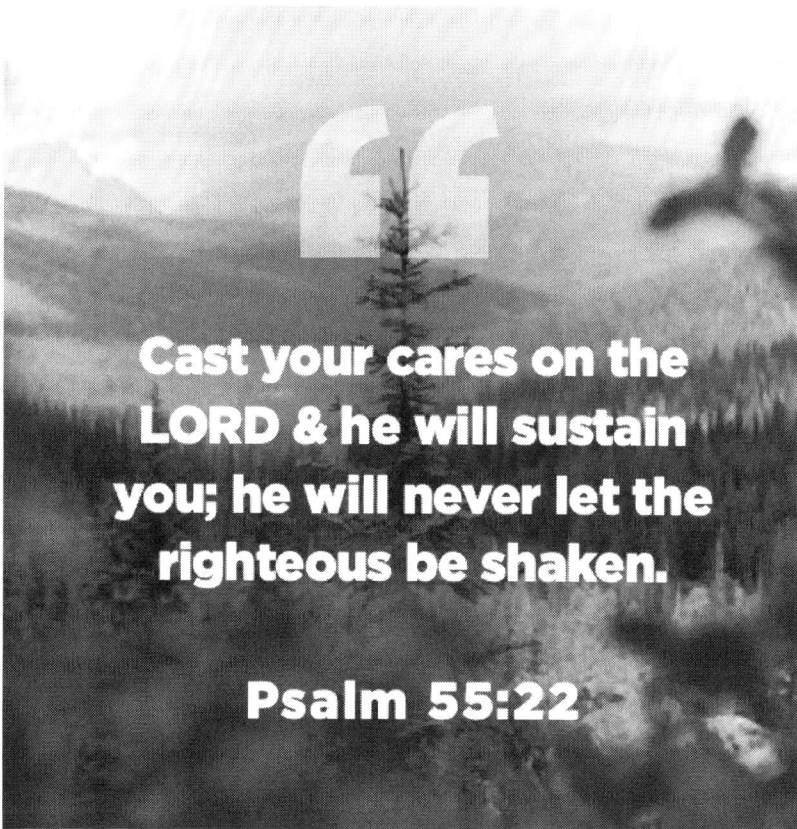

> **Cast your cares on the LORD & he will sustain you; he will never let the righteous be shaken.**
>
> **Psalm 55:22**

God's power, His dynamite, his atomic bomb, is love. Loving an individual like me, in such a way that I am reassured, comforted, seen clearly, known intimately, healed at the core of my being, set on a high rock so I can continue in my purpose. That is love like a supernova, and it's available to us all, every day. I didn't realize I was fighting that love because my definition contained self-sufficiency that was put there by me, not Him.

I added a prayer for others going through chemo, people who were in my infusion center during my visits, people whose illness was shared with me in several different ways, from friends, family, and social media. I developed prayers to cover the specifics of cancer and prayed for the complete healing of others every day. Below is a healing prayer against cancer that can be used by individuals or groups to pray for one another:

In the name of Jesus, I (we) command that (person's name) cancer be destroyed at the root, never to return, that the root of cancer in (person's name) body leave now, in the name of Jesus. I declare in Jesus's name that all cancer and side effects of cancer and cancer treatments will never harm (person's name). I command that (person's name) DNA, their body chemistry and genetics change now to conform to God's original intention, His original design for them. I declare that Jesus is restoring to (person's name) everything they lost, and He always restores to a place greater than before; so now (person's name) has greater health, greater well-being, and wellness. In Jesus's name. Amen.

While I hung out on my couch, my family was there for me every day; they behaved as if doing absolutely nothing for an entire week was a natural thing; no complaints or suggestions. They didn't miss a beat. They taught me so much about what support looks like. We watched movies, sports, and sports and movies as if it was something normal. I decided to learn how to blog, so while I laid on the couch eating my 15th lifesaver because lifesavers were all I could eat, I taught myself how to blog and set up a site. Anything to feel like I could still contribute, could still be a part of God's plan for something. Even in this state, there were more positives than negatives, and I felt God blessing me and preparing me for His service one day.

I only had two good days before Chemo #4, but they were filled with powerful insights. I was convinced that God would never mismanage my life. I chose to live above my circumstances because that is what allowed the power of God to work in me and on my behalf. The understanding was dawning in my mind that I could declare the exact opposite of what I was experiencing as truth in my life; that where I placed my belief was my choice and the source of my power and victory.

So I praised God during my worst bouts of nausea, I would pray for the nurses while they were putting on protective gear prior to popping the infusion bag to begin the course of treatment that was the most toxic, and I praised God as I white knuckled my keyboard while trying to string together a coherent sentence at work while chemo tried to scramble my brain.

I reasoned that, as soon as I became a believer, persecution came—physically, and financially—but I viewed persecution as proof that God had a good plan for my life, so good and true that the devil would try every deceit to make me lose heart and turn away from my blessing and my purpose. But that was never going to happen, so all he was doing was creating debt for himself that will need to be repaid to me. I fought the devil every day by speaking life, speaking the Word over my life, and refusing to despair and believe his lies, like this:

In the name of Jesus, I declare and decree that the devil's ability to inflict me with loss is over. My debts will be paid, and my health fully restored by Christmas. I declare the devil is a thief and has been caught stealing from me, and I release my faith over Proverbs 6:31: And if the thief is caught, he must pay back seven-fold, even up to the whole substance of his house. Devil, you are caught. I will never stop crying for justice and my jury is God Almighty, Jesus His Son, and The Holy Spirit. I will gladly show others how to operate as children of Abraham, children of the covenant of God, capable of performing signs, wonders, miracles, and things greater than these because Jesus went to the Father (John 14:12-14). And I will continue to preach the gospel, heal the sick and pray for others every day I am on this earth. Jesus said in John 10:18: No one can take my life from me. I sacrifice it voluntarily. I have the authority to lay it down when I want to and also to take it up again. For this is what my Father has commanded. So, I declare that I do not lay down my life for another 60 years at least!

I kept up with my list of everything that was stolen from me by the devil, including:

- ❖ Time with my family
- ❖ Health
- ❖ Peace
- ❖ Relationships
- ❖ Money
- ❖ Property
- ❖ Patience
- ❖ Jobs
- ❖ Security
- ❖ Laughter

All must be paid back sevenfold according to the Word of God, which is the sword I used for battle. I spoke this aloud and added dollars wherever I could. As in, "devil, you stole my paid-off car from me, that's $20,000 that has to be paid back sevenfold."

The devil cannot win. He has already lost. Christ won over 2,000 years ago and He expects me, expects all of us who believe in Him, to live as if He won. As if we are winners. Amen and amen.

20

CHEMO #4

A MIRACLE SAVE

I was apprehensive about this one because chemo #3 was so challenging, but I finally drew up in front of the line at the pharmacy to refill my meds, when I was told, "I'm sorry, we no longer carry your insurance." I was stunned and waves of panic began to wash over me as I considered what it would mean to complete my treatments without insurance.

One infusion alone was thousands of dollars…

Wait…

Stop…

This is another negative, another attack, another test.

I calmed down, thanked the pharmacist I had for eight years, and drove away.

I went to a second pharmacy and spoke with a very nice woman who told me that just that month, they started carrying my insurance provider. She had also beaten cancer five years earlier.

Two hours later, I not only had my meds in hand, but the protocol for taking them was printed right on the bottle. For the last three infusions, the pharmacy said the protocol was too long to print out. They provided a handwritten note with directions, but I never saw the note and threw out the pharmacy bag every time.

As I read the instructions on the bottle, I realized that for my last treatments, I had been dosing myself incorrectly. As a result, I had been shorting my meds every treatment and compounding the toxic levels that were accumulating for the next treatment—no wonder I was feeling so bad!

God knew what was happening and recognized that three times I ignored the instructions, so the only way to get through to me was to change pharmacies so I would get the right instructions and dosage for Chemo #4. And bonus, the prescription was completely free!

Thank You, Father, for Your care and concern and working miracles in the lives of your children! Amen and Amen!

Chemo #4 was a respite; I turned the corner in three days and with only two more infusions to go, the light at the end of the tunnel was growing brighter. I began noticing more and more people beating cancer. I believed we were learning about the power we have as Christians to heal others and ourselves. I believed we were overcoming cancer with healing prayers, decrees, and declarations. That as a big single biomass we were ourselves turning the corner and beginning to heal.

One of the things I heard regularly about healing was that after being healed, I should do something, try something that was out of the ordinary for someone who was "sick," thereby showing my faith in my healing. I am not, repeat *not*, recommending this to others, but I do want to share my story. I attended a sales call on the west coast and flew there to be in person. This meant exposing myself, during chemo, to the highest risk of all, which is being around other people. On an airplane, which is a petri dish with wings. I stayed with family, not in a hotel, so some risk was minimized, but I'm sure I had my share of exposure to…whatever, just plenty of exposure.

Years later, when I think of that sales call, I am so thankful that the person I met with didn't register shock when I appeared, with a beanie on my head that I never took off, no apparent hair, face all puffy from chemo, no eyebrows except for some I was trying to create with makeup, and my crazy Vegas eyelashes. He acted as if everything was completely normal and I felt like a person again, regardless of my appearance. It was a positive step, and one I will always be thankful for.

I was studying Pastor Jerry Savelle, and by this time I felt like the Holy Spirit's student; my curriculum came from Him regularly. There was no syllabus or outline to give me a big picture of what we were doing together or what would come next, but I made choices about the material to spend time with that felt guided, and once I dove into a subject, it became clear why.

The subject was breakthroughs, and I felt the need to be prepared for one. While the topic itself was compelling, when I came across his teaching about offense, I was convicted and knew I needed to pay attention.

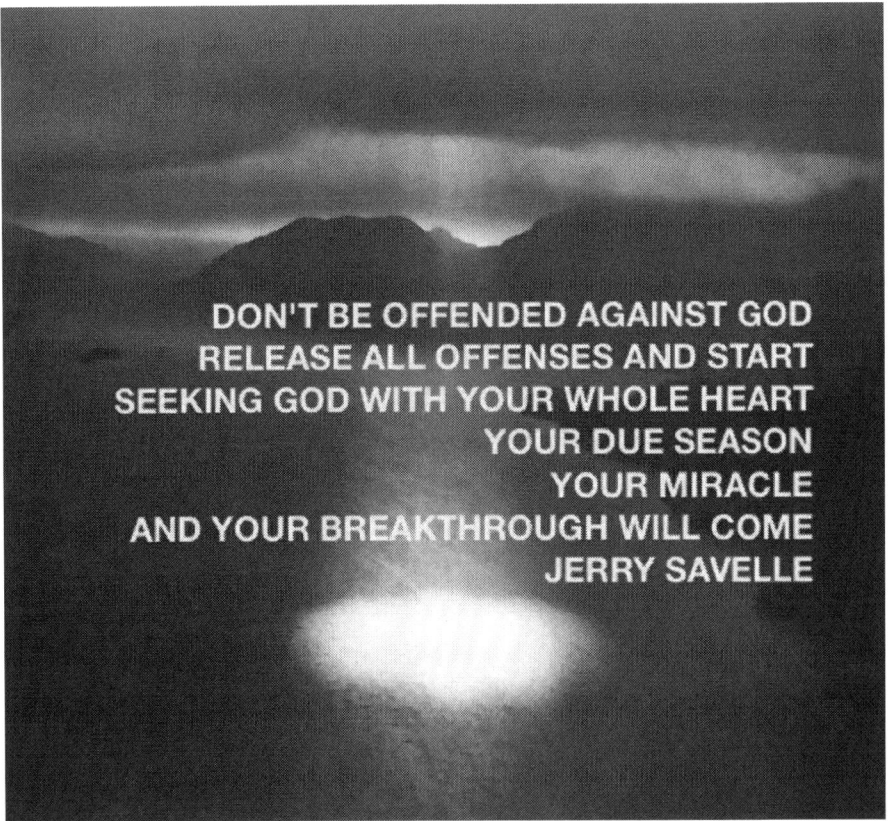

DON'T BE OFFENDED AGAINST GOD
RELEASE ALL OFFENSES AND START
SEEKING GOD WITH YOUR WHOLE HEART
YOUR DUE SEASON
YOUR MIRACLE
AND YOUR BREAKTHROUGH WILL COME
JERRY SAVELLE

Release all offenses; I could not get my mind off that phrase. I had started a practice of calligraphy in my work notebooks; I would write a phrase the Holy Spirit called out for me in my daily calendar so I would see it throughout the week and keep it in mind. Release all offenses. It came across to me as proactive and all-encompassing. Release, as in don't consider the offense, or study the offense or have a discussion about the offense, just let it go, now. All of them, not some of them, not just the ones that are petty or only affecting me in a minor way, but all of them. It took me two weeks of attention to this phrase, sifting through memories, along with the immediate, daily opportunities to be offended, to feel that I was making headway.

The mindset to release all offenses had to be ever-present because the temptation to be offended was a 24/7 guarantee as long as we are alive and living on this planet.

Offense is another lie straight from Satan. It appears justifiable, self-righteous, wholly understandable, yet it is a toxin, a poison that hurts the offended, not the offender.

The Holy Spirit asked, "Would you go out every morning looking for heavy rocks to put in your pockets, your bag, your backpack, just keep loading yourself up with rocks and carrying that weight, all the while telling yourself that someone else was carrying it?"

Because that's what offense is—a big, heavy rock, some heavier than others, that I picked up, that I chose to carry, that I chose to accumulate and allowed to weigh me down, that did not affect anyone else but me. Why did I do that? I pictured myself emptying my pockets, my purse, and my backpack, of all the rocks I was carrying. And when the temptation to become offended happens now, which it does every single day and often many times in a day, I see it for the rock that it is, and I do not pick it up. I am weightless and free, in the name of Jesus.

Chemo #5 was near and I was starting the side effect meds. Only two more infusions to go. I was feeling so good, may I never take for granted what it feels like to exist without pain and discomfort. The mind game that chemo plays is about the reality of the moment. I was reveling in feeling normal, but the closer I came to the infusion date, the more apprehensive I would be because I knew I wouldn't feel normal again at some point.

The apprehension affected my ability to enjoy the time I felt well, and I wanted to overcome that anxiety.

I knew that 1 John 4:18 says, "There is no fear in love, but perfect love casts out fear because fear involves torment. But he who fears has not been made perfect in love."

I decided to replace the word love with faith, because fear is a form of energy in search of a negative outcome and faith is its opposite, a form of energy in search of a positive outcome.

THE PRAYING MEDIC SAYS IT BEST:

When we fear the return of sickness, we do so because we doubt that God has really healed us or that we will remain healed. We may also doubt that He truly loves us. Fear and doubt about God's goodness allow the enemy to bring sickness back. When we live from a place of faith, we walk on ground that God has given us as our possession. It is our inheritance and our refuge. Faith is our place of strength.

The enemy is at a disadvantage when we walk on the ground called faith.

When we walk in doubt and fear, we walk on the enemy's ground, which allows him to keep us in pain.

Where we walk is a choice we have to make. The choice we make determines the outcome of our healing.

Fear will keep us in sickness.

Faith will keep us healed. This is why we must close our account with sickness and choose never again to entertain these thoughts.

I chose to live in the now, the moment during which I was healed, during which I had no pain, and to deny satan the ability to deceive me into living anything other than joyful. I practiced taking deep breaths and imagining Jesus stretching time out with his hands, from a portrait to a panoramic view of my moment, and holding it there until I was ready to take the next breath, praising Him while my anxiety floated away like a cloud.

During this time, in 2017, I had the opportunity to pray, along with many others, for a young woman recently diagnosed with Stage 4 pancreatic cancer. Today, nearly 3 years later, she is alive and well.

Prayers lift us up, and distance prayers are just as effective as those prayed in the presence of the individual.

HERE IS ONE YOU CAN USE ANYWHERE, ANYTIME:

FATHER, IN THE NAME OF JESUS CHRIST OF NAZARETH WHOM I SERVE, WE DECLARE THAT ALL TRAUMA, CANCER, SIDE EFFECTS FROM CANCER TREATMENTS, ALL ILLNESS, INFIRMITY, AND LACK LEAVE [NAME] NOW. AND THAT JESUS HIMSELF WOULD RESTORE EVERYTHING THAT WAS STOLEN FROM HER. HE IS THE GOD OF RESTORATION AND ALWAYS RESTORES TO A PLACE GREATER THAN BEFORE. WE DECREE COMPLETE HEALING AND RESTORATION OVER HER BODY, HER SPIRIT, HER FAMILY AND HER FINANCES. WE DECLARE [NAME] IS NOW WELL, PHYSI-CALLY, SPIRITUALLY AND FINANCIALLY, AND SHE IS RESTORED TO HER FAMILY, HER FUTURE AND HER DESTINY IN CHRIST.
IN THE MIGHTY NAME OF JESUS, AMEN AND AMEN.

My place in the world of healing seemed to be more about prayers, praying for others and showing others how to pray. I wasn't certain about it yet, but I kept my written prayers along with the prayers of others I felt the Holy Spirit pointing out to me.

21

Chemo #5

Strike Amidships

On day eight after chemo #5, I experienced a bout of respiratory and stomach flu. I burned my hand on a hot pan. My checking account was overdrawn, which meant I went out to two banks, while sick, to fix it. And all this happened during a two-day flash flood watch in my neighborhood. I knew I was getting the full attack and readied my mind to fight back.

My little girl, whose school was the source of the stomach flu, succumbed to it herself first. She came home from school, said her stomach hurt and within 10 minutes was projectile vomiting on the couch, the floor, and herself. I was the only one home, and I'm her mom, so my response needed to be about her, not about the likely next phase in this process for me due to the exposure I experienced cleaning up after her. Based on the place I was in the chemo cycle, my immune system was flat on its back on the mat and the referee had already yelled out two counts. I praised God that I could be there for her and just be the mom that she needed then.

A few hours later, after everyone was in bed, I was in the basement when it hit me. I retched in every available sink in my house, erping my way back upstairs and camping out in the living room for the night. And I praised Jesus. Lying on the couch, quarantined from my husband, staring at Conan O'Brian and trying not to wake the family with my heaving, I raised my hands and praised Him. Never before have I praised my Jesus when the current reality was so obviously not in my favor. Because satan was trying to see if I would give up, if I would retract my former statements about the goodness of God, and because God wanted me strengthened. He wanted to make certain that my resolve, my belief in Him no matter what, was rock solid. That when tested, I would come forth as gold.

And so I praised you, Jesus, still reeling, imagining I would never eat again, shuffling from the couch to the bathroom like a 90-year-old, I praised You. There was victory in my praise! I declared Romans 4:17 over my life that day, "who calls that which is not as though it were."

I laid on the couch, the light of the laptop shining off the top of my bald head like some kind of full moon taking place in the living room, and read Joel 2:21-27 over and over again. It was the only thing that made me feel like me again and not the alien from Mars. And that was the greatest miracle; that I could be in the state I was, alone, searching for the word that would accurately de-

124

scribe how sick I was, but I was not frightened. I did not panic, I had peace.

What God tries to tell us and the Holy Spirit tries to demonstrate is that focusing on Him, praising Him, is not an exercise in perfect righteousness, it is not some supreme adoration or acknowledging God's superiority while heaving, it is a method for strengthening our emotional response to an awful situation so that we can be whole as we deal with it by speaking overcoming words. To praise God when I did not have anything at the moment to praise about but to praise anyway was overcoming language that righted, supported, and calmed my mind and emotions.

It took what could have been, what the devil wanted it to be, a night of defeat, and turned it into….just a Thursday night that my kid came home sick and passed it along to me. It took the crappiness of cleaning up after an award-winning blast of stomach flu and turned it into my ability to show my daughter that I could still be her mom by doing the things that mattered. And it became a memory of my ability to run again to God instead of away from Him when things got tough.

Because being the hero of your own life means standing up to whatever tries to take you down. It means remembering your training as a human being, as a follower of Christ, because your kids are watching, and this life lesson is critical.

Satan, you are nothing but a bully and the entire world has had enough of you. You use cancer to pick on children, mothers, and fathers. You think that your evil will erode our trust in God, that you can deceive us into thinking, "how could God allow our babies, our husbands, and wives, our grandparents, to suffer from this?" But you are a liar and the father of lies because God wouldn't allow it. He gave us the ability to heal by faith, and we need to stand up and take the mantle and fight! Jesus said in John 14:12-13:

Truly, truly, I tell you, whoever believes in Me will also do the works that I am doing. He will do even greater things than these, because I am going to the Father. And I will do whatever you ask in My name, so that the Father may be glorified in the Son.

Jesus was telling us that, as believers, we are supposed to handle cancer, not let cancer handle us. I am convinced this is one of the reasons Jesus said in Matthew 17:17-18: "O unbelieving and perverse generation! Jesus replied. "How long must I remain with you? How long must I put up with you? Bring the boy here to Me." Then Jesus rebuked the demon, and it came out of the boy, and he was healed from that moment.

Perhaps He was frustrated because we are supposed to step up into our covenant rights and responsibilities and do something ourselves.

Jesus, I am asking in your name for the mantle to destroy cancer and the current cures in my lifetime. To take away its ability to steal, destroy and kill. To turn it from a dragon into a kitten with no ability to hurt, ever again. No more radiation or chemo poison for people. No more excruciating biopsies, ports in our bodies, surgical maiming or watching our children, our parents, our spouses, and friends suffer.

Cancer is about fear, but perfect love casts out fear. Perfect love, the kind that says, I'm scared, but I'm not giving my attention and everything precious about my life to some worn out devil that already lost the battle and is sticking around to see how many innocent people he can make as miserable as he is.

In the name of Jesus Christ of Nazareth, whom I serve, I declare cancer's ability to destroy, steal and end lives is over.

After not one but two bouts of the flu, my immune system slowly, doggedly, returned. Like Rocky in the last round, buoyed by the knowledge that there was only one more round to go, my spirits lifted as I felt my body rally. The light in my heart was still there, doing a slow burn, but I knew, I knew it would never go out. I experienced peace and praise in the middle of chaos and focused on my family, work, and getting some calories before the next infusion.

I was watching a video series titled, "The Truth About Cancer." It was a 9+-hour documentary that covered research about causes, treatments, and resources for cancer patients and their families. I went back into student mode, spending one and a half hours each night watching, taking notes, and reviewing the research on my own. This is a very distilled summarization, but I learned some basics about the scientific research:

Cancer is a symptom, not a cause. Cancer can be telling you the immune system is under stress and needs support. Think about things that are consistently impacting you and your body, through daily activities like eating, drinking, managing pain and stress, anything that requires the immune system to fire up and expend resources to provide support. The idea is that the immune system has a finite capability to fight intrusions; so managing the accumulated impact is the goal. If there is an area where you can't limit exposure, try to limit the overall impact by reducing exposure somewhere else. Some examples include:

1. Heavy metal poisoning – fillings in your teeth can be a cause of consistent stress on the immune system. Certain fish are heavy metal targets, canned tuna and salmon that aren't wild-caught, for example. If you eat these types of fish with a high rate of regularity, there is an immune system impact.

2. Water that you drink – daily intake of water that is chlorinated, has fluoride and other "small" doses of chemicals requires the immune system to engage and counteract the toxins. There are many water filtration systems available that operate at the source (prior to coming out of your faucet) or that filter water out of your faucet through everything as simple as a water pitcher with a filter to an onboard filtration system in your refrigerator.

3. The acidity of your system – the pH of your system can be out of balance due to high acid foods and drinks. Bottled water is readily available that is pH balanced, or you can research the use of apple cider vinegar.

4. Magnetic frequency – the earth has a magnetic frequency that harmonizes cell activity and deactivates free radicals. Things that disrupt the frequency create an environment that allows cancer to flourish. Constant exposure to cell phones, especially held up against the head, impacts the immune system. I use headsets and the speaker on the phone rather than hold the phone up to my head, and I try to limit my screen time. This is one of the toughest things for me to do based on my work, so I double down on limiting the immune system impact in other areas to make up for it.

5. Food – I limit my intake of processed foods by reading labels and staying as close to raw as I can. Processed foods include chemicals and the body has to process them like toxins, which impacts the immune system. If an ingredient label has more than 5 ingredients and includes chemical names, I put it back on the shelf. I stopped eating refined sugar, and limit high acid foods. I also support my immune system with green tea, at least one cup and often two or three cups a day, especially when I travel.

6. Stress and pain – constant chronic stress in your body. The source of stress could be emotional, financial, physical (chronic pain causes inflammation and a stress response) which impacts the immune system. Don't ignore chronic pain as this can cause a cascading health problem. If you suffer from chronic pain, continue to seek healing. Research healers who have healed others of chronic pain and email them, watch them on

YouTube, find out if they are ever in your area, or would recommend someone for your physical issue. Don't give up until you have found someone who can help you, or keep healing yourself on your own until it works!

What I learned is that if there is something that is constantly provoking an immune system response, it places stress on the immune system and makes it hard for it to find and destroy pre-cancerous cells. Normally the immune system finds and destroys cancer or pre-cancerous cells every day like no big deal, but when the immune system is weak, cancer cells can multiply beyond the immune system's ability to destroy them.

This is an extremely abridged version of a complex health problem. I encourage you to do your research and reach your conclusions, which ultimately will guide you to your healing. The Holy Spirit will help you! James 4:2 says, "you do not have because you do not ask God." So ask! All day, every day, ask for what you need. He will be there and He will show you the next step to take. Just ask and listen.

22

CHEMO #6

DANTE'S CIRCLE OF HELL

That seems dramatic, but it's how the experience panned out and it was entirely about nausea. Nausea. A circle of hell that traps you by somehow making you think it will never end. The experience prevents any notion of a bigger picture, an end game. And while I struggled to manage it, my body starved for calories I couldn't take in. I'm sure there is a Greek drama to illustrate my frustration with being so insanely hungry I would quickly stuff a single bite of sandwich or pasta in my mouth, only to have it turn to moldy ashes and bring on waves of illness before I could swallow it.

Leave it to satan to create a situation where a double mastectomy is more appealing than another round of chemo. But that's where I was; back in the surgeon's office, where I was told that the tumor was still there (was the earlier doctor conducting placebo research? Why did he say that to me?) and had broken off into some lymph nodes, so things needed to happen quickly.

But my prayer life! God told me repeatedly I was not going to have surgery. He gave me a rhema word—Let Me Do This For You—and I submitted gratefully, having no idea how to manage the next phase of my treatment, especially since I could barely navigate breakfast. He was going to work a powerful miracle in my life, and I praised Him. Father, thank You for this encouragement. Today, I stand under the open windows of heaven and praise You for Your blessings. Amen and Amen! I continued to encourage myself with online videos from Joel Osteen and Joyce Meyer. I watched healing and spiritual videos daily; they provided peace and strengthened me. Like a force field, they surrounded me with hope and protection.

Because I would never have it again, chemo #6 quickly became a distant memory, but my body was holding fluids and my hands and face were still puffy. I asked my oncologist about some ways to detox after chemo and he referred me to another physician on the team. About a week later I met with him and asked about detoxing and he cut me off and demanded that I sit down at the computer in the examining room and tell him "where on the internet I had found any real research" about the need to detox my body. He became immediately angry and condescending and kept pointing to the chair in front of the keyboard, telling me, "sit down and show me—come on, show me!" He was in instant attack mode, and I was shocked at first, telling him that it was logical to me that after six rounds of highly toxic chemical compounds, my liver might need some support; that the cancer cells destroyed by the chemo might exit my body faster somehow, and my goal was to support my body. What could be wrong with seeking a medical opinion about that?

Again, his response was angry, confrontational and patronizing. He didn't share his research or provide a logical counterpoint to my concerns; he told me I knew nothing and had no basis for my questions. He said there "was nothing I could do and nothing I needed to do except drink water." I took a deep breath and did something I had never done before. I told him, "this appointment is over. I'm the one who is fighting this battle, and it's my body. I came here for help, not to be yelled at or talked down to. We are done here. Thank you for your time." And I walked. Calmly, with my bald head and the last vestiges of my eyebrows and Vegas eyelashes, I walked.

Father, I learned something that day. Up until that point, I had complete trust in my doctors and the team of medical people who worked with me. Which wasn't wrong, but wasn't right, either. My body, my health, and my healing were my responsibility, and I acknowledged that truth. I felt an awareness within that felt amazingly like joy, joy that came from calmly standing up for myself in a situation meant to negatively influence me. And I didn't own any of the behavior or emotional outbursts I had just witnessed. I didn't internalize it or try to work through it. I rejected the entire scene like it was something out of a movie. I had enough going on in my life at that moment and chose to forgive the offense and move on.

I learned many things during the illness, especially from that awkward, confrontational scene in the doctor's office. First, my body was my responsibility and I had a right to my concerns and to seek guidance wherever my research led me. Second, that I would never again own the emotional response of someone else. I would listen, try to understand, forgive and shed the experience. When it comes to negativity in any form, I learned that I needed to travel light.

When my oncologist asked me how the appointment went, I told him I was disappointed and felt the doctor was the least like a physician that I had encountered so far, but that the experience drove me to contend for my healing, which was a good thing; a God thing. That I found some simple things I could do that I felt helped my body cleanse itself; matcha tea and daily wheatgrass shots. Simple. And I moved on to the next phase of the process—surgery.

23

EVERYTHING IS HEADED IN THE RIGHT DIRECTION

I had post-chemo mammograms and went to my oncologist for the results. When my husband asked her what the results showed, she would only repeat, "everything is headed in the right direction." At the time, I thought this meant that the tumor was gone and the lymph node that had been infected with the disease was clear. That was when we learned that the typical protocol for cancer is two-pronged at least; in my case, just having chemo wouldn't be enough. We then discussed the oncologist's recommendation: a lumpectomy and radiation.

My husband and I discussed this. They found some "probably" benign tissue in my right breast as well as the small tumor in my left. Our decision was a double mastectomy. Our daughter is 8 years old. I am 56. Take them both and let's go. The doctor's first comment was, "well, that's fine, but this will take about 2 years to accomplish." When I asked why, she asked, "Well, you'll want them bigger, right?" We both stared at her and said, "NO! This is not a pitch for free breast enhancement surgery!" She then conceded that, if I didn't want bigger breasts, they could do the mastectomy and the implants/reconstruction at the same time. I would be golfing again in 6 weeks and able to walk/run my first week after surgery.

We set up a time for the surgery, got the name of the plastic surgeon I needed to meet with, and ended the appointment. The next day as I was doing my devotions, I was spending time with God, asking Him if He had a word for me. Was there any direction He wanted to give me, something I could do or follow for Him? He immediately said, "You will not have this surgery."

LET ME DO THIS FOR YOU. DO NOT LIMIT ME. LET ME LOVE YOU. LET OTHER PEOPLE LOVE YOU.

I cried as I processed why it was so, so hard for me to do that, how root cause that information was for me. As a child, I learned early that I would have to fend for myself, and once that became apparent, my mode of operation, my go-to strategy for life, the only approach that kept me from panicking on a regular basis, was to strive, strive, strive to take care of myself. I doubled down to figure things out and protect myself, even to judge and condemn myself when things over which I truly had no control happened, because at least then I could still maintain a sense of single-handed cause and effect. I couldn't let other people love me because I couldn't trust anyone, period.

So now what? God was asking me to trust Him, but He was also saying He would do it for me. That in the future, whenever I was asked about my healing, I would always say that God did it. Because He did. My answer was, "Lord, I trust You and that is a monumental submission for me. I trust you, I will let You do this for me; I will not limit you. I will let You and others love me." Peace followed. But not for long.

Daily, my peace was attacked. My work in sales began to flounder in ridiculous ways. Deals fell apart, one after another, leaving me with drastically reduced income and a team that was shell shocked from the experience of daily losses. I received my scans and learned that my lymph node was clear, and the tumor itself had shrunk a tiny bit but was still there. Still there. STILL THERE. Ok, so I am carrying on with my thinking that God will heal me, that He has already healed me, but I still have a plastic surgeon meeting, the date for my surgery is 22 days away, and the blasted tumor is still in me.

My family would not support me in saying no to the surgery. God's word was repeated daily.

LET ME DO THIS FOR YOU. DO NOT PLACE LIMITS ON ME.

The difference between what was taking place in my life naturally vs. supernaturally was extremely stressful, but by spending time with some form of God's Word, I could finally achieve peace and replace negative thoughts with scripture. This sounds simple, but it was not. It was a daily battle, and I cannot stress enough that it was daily. Every. Day.

Only in hindsight do I understand the critical lesson I learned about placing my trust in God that was a direct result of those four weeks of laboring to maintain peace regardless of the chaos and attacks that surrounded me. I want to be clear that the process was not easy but the outcome each day was positive and the alternatives were worse.

Achieving and maintaining my peace did not mean I never cried or experienced depression, anger, frustration, and loss. It meant that I viewed those feelings and emotions as temporary situations from which I grew more and more able to move through and move on from. Negative emotions are not something to avoid at all costs; they were a necessary part of the process of change I found myself dealing with. But I learned that I could give them a virtual nod of the head, acknowledge their existence, and keep moving. I intuitively knew that passing through those emotional phases was unavoidable, but staying too long in those emotional states would impact my healing.

It's also true that people, normally kind people, wildly successful, uber educated people, even the people closest to you, are not perfect and most do not handle catastrophic illness well. I had people rush up to me to recount their stories of family members who died from cancer. I had to acknowledge the cleverness of satan during these times. Like Wile E. Coyote, he would pop up in the form of another person saying something completely inappropriate to me.

Many, many people have been wounded by cancer in their lives and never processed their loss because they weren't the victim. When they saw me with the telltale beanie on my head, they were thrown into emotional pain and used me to process through it or relive it. I chose to help them process through it rather than take offense.

Paul says in Ephesians 6:12:

For we wrestle not against flesh and blood, but against principalities, against powers, against the rulers of the darkness of this world, against spiritual wickedness in high places.

I saw evidence of this truth especially when well-meaning people said the wrong things to me; when doctors misunderstood my intentions and when strangers made assumptions about my condition. In these instances, it was clear to me that Wile E. Coyote was the culprit, not the individual. I would smile and ask them to tell me more about their story; I would comfort where I could. When attacked, as I was by the doctor, I calmly thanked him for his time and ended the appointment. My goal was to throw love around where satan tried to cause pain.

In her book, *Undaunted*, Christine Caine, upon learning as an adult that she had been adopted at birth, says: What was I going to do? …Love, I thought. I am going to love others like I never had before. This approach resonated with my spirit in a way that helped pull me through negativity and refocused me. To love others, to love on them, to desire to help them, to do the opposite of what you feel when experiencing negativity, is one of the most powerful ways to fight illness.

To do this acknowledges the way the world should work; not the way it's working at that particular moment, but how you know it should work. It pulls heaven down to earth. Satan may be able to orchestrate negativity through people, but God gave us the ability to orchestrate heaven ourselves from within and we have the opportunity to do that every day.

I learned from an essay by Bill Johnson in his book, *Essentials of Healing*, that it could be that God was allowing me to go through the process in this manner because He knew I would recognize His signal to believe, to hang on, to trust, to go deeper into His Word for support, and ultimately achieve a greater victory than I could have on my own, something that would ultimately benefit others and glorify Himself in a more meaningful way.

I had some days when this all made sense to me and some days when all I wanted was my golf swing back; to play with my daughter and have no more battles with fear, no more attacks on me and my family. I would imagine how Abraham felt leading Isaac to the sacrificial altar, not telling him the real reason for the trip. I couldn't blast out to my family and friends that yep, still had the tumor, but nope, wasn't having the surgery! I could only walk the walk of faith and know that somehow God was going to resolve this in my favor as long as I would submit to Him and place no limits on Him.

Daily I would work to "pray myself into peace." Some days that took minutes, some days it took hours. Romans 4:17, to call things that aren't as though they are, became my mantra. Then I abandoned it because it felt as if I was declaring that things AREN'T when I already knew that they WERE. I just read scripture, read books about healing, read books about the Holy Spirit and words of knowledge until my panic went away.

And ultimately, I got to the place where I stopped panicking when deals fell apart. I led the team differently because I stopped freaking out when things went wrong. On the inside, I was still shaking my head, but honestly, it got to be predictable. And yet, the Word said victory was mine; peace was mine; joy was mine. So I started living in joy even as my circumstances appeared negative in the natural.

Here is an example of a reading that would calm my spirit. This is from Bev Robinson. All praise to You, Father!

Ready yourself. Let Me fill your body, soul and spirit with faith. You will soon move up, into another realm of blessing. This has been preparing to come for quite some time, and the time is drawing near now. When the faith comes, do not give unbelief the time of day. Resist it at all costs. I will show you what to do. Fill your mind with My word. Fill your thoughts and emotions with faith. Resist unbelief.

Hebrews 11:1 (NLT): "Faith is the confidence that what we hope for will actually happen; it gives us assurance about things we cannot see."

So I am nine days out from surgery day, and I stopped at the Miracle House to let them know what was going on. They referred me to a Novena of Surrender to help me submit my will to God in this matter.

The Novena is below. It is a nine-day Novena! This should come as no surprise to me. I'm starting to get used to miracles on a daily and sometimes hourly basis.

Thank you, Father, for your kindness to me and your wonders to the sons of men!

Father Don Dolindo Ruotolo wrote this Novena of Surrender to the Will of God.

The link[1] is below, but Day 7 spoke most clearly to me:

---

[1]

https://www.catholicdoors.com/prayers/novenas/p03530.htm

I perform miracles in proportion to your full surrender to me
and to your not thinking of yourselves.
I sow treasure troves of graces
when you are in the deepest poverty.
No person of reason, no thinker,
has ever performed miracles,
not even among the saints.
He does divine works whosoever surrenders to God.
So don't think about it any more,
because your mind is acute
and for you it is very hard to see evil
and to trust in me
and to not think of yourself.
Do this for all your needs,
do this all of you
and you will see great continual silent miracles.
I will take care of things,
I promise this to you.
(Repeat the following prayer 10 times.)
O Jesus, I surrender myself to you,
take care of everything!

God continues to direct me daily. I have learned how to be alert, how to watch, listen and be obedient to His leading. A week ago, I listened to a Joel Osteen video, during which he said, "Go to the house of the Lord."

I knew the message was for me, and I had attended a book study at church on Saturday and service on Sunday. That Sunday was communion, something I had wanted to take for months, and the congregation was offered healing and I found myself covered by healing prayer and petitions.

During the process, my body heated up, and I'm certain healing happened to me. The pastor anointed me, and she and another member prayed over me a second time. The pastor told me that I should consider if there was any unforgiveness or bitterness in my heart towards anyone and if so, just ask God to reveal it and help me let it go. The second lady said she felt God told her to share with me that I needed to keep believing what He told me, to resist unbelief.

24

UNFORGIVENESS

As I was receiving prayer for healing, the two ladies praying for me shared that 1) I should stay strong and keep believing what God told me and 2) I should consider if there is anyone I need to forgive, because sometimes the root of cancer is unforgiveness and bitterness. As He had done in the past, the Holy Spirit illuminated these thoughts in my mind and I knew I needed to consider their words.

Everyone has a "tree of life" with fruit they need to stay away from. An area of potential weakness that God wants to heal and redeem and satan wants to control and exploit to steal, kill and destroy. The key is focus. Satan was able to exploit Eve and Adam's weakness to get them to focus on the one thing they didn't have versus all the blessings God had bestowed freely on them.

And he tried to do this with me, too. In my case, I was open to moving my focus off of all God had done for me when I perceived I had been wronged. Unforgiveness is one of my areas of weakness. Unforgiveness, judgment, and bitterness had become a trifecta of focus for me until I realized the game he was playing with me, and how easily I fell for it.

The more I thought about it, I realized that there was a pattern to the process of being unforgiving, a way that it worked in my life to undermine my attitude and steal my joy. I judged myself daily. What God meant for discernment, the ability to see people and situations through His eyes, had become a painful process of comparison and failure through mine. The more I failed at life, the more I judged others and myself.

But failure is so misunderstood in our culture, and when I forced myself to face my failures—a failed marriage, lost business, relationships that had ended, times when I was so disappointed in my behavior—the list could go on and on, as I had become an astute scribe for my life's fiascoes. I learned two things. I had made mistakes, yes, but when I spoke with others about them, people who had been around me virtually all my life, they remembered things differently. Not to say that I wasn't wrong, or that I couldn't have done things differently, but that I had crystallized moments of my personal history into drops of pure, focused guilt that was unnecessary and unhealthy, primarily because I never let them go. I wore them like a jeweled necklace everywhere I went. I had accepted Christ, acknowledged that he died for every foolish, wrong, hurtful, embarrassing thing I had ever done, but I still put that necklace on every day. If anyone had asked me, I would have told them that, of course, I forgave myself, but I had no grace for myself, and so had no grace for others.

I viewed this penchant for distilling my behavior as a side effect of perfectionism. And while I knew that perfectionism is the opposite of grace, it was a hard habit for me to break because it gave me a sense of control that I felt I needed to survive. But there are a host of complications that are born out of perfectionism that had grown like weeds in my thinking and then my heart. That necklace didn't just memorialize my failures, it provided lenses through which I constantly interpreted other people and situations, like a string of different magnifying crystals that was immediately available for me to use to judge others.

The Holy Spirit showed me that perfectionism is key to thinking patterns based on control and image management. When people need to be perfect, they must also have control. But the world often doesn't allow that to work one hundred percent of the time; so what's the answer? Especially if you are five, seven, nine years old and have no support or role models close at hand? Expend energy building and maintaining an image of control. It's not real, but if you can convince yourself and the people around you that it is, you've made progress, and progress in those situations is literally just making it through another day looking as if you actually understand and can manage what's going on around you.

This is the antithesis of trusting God for an outcome, but it's often used as a method for survival in people who struggle with a loss of trust and self-image as a child, and it worked for me. Not the best approach, but there are millions of children whose situations require that they fight for themselves during their youth. With limited skills and tools, they do the best they can. Fake it until you make it and somewhere in that process, you'll learn to be who you think you should be. Except that when I got there, I didn't have a sense of my own authenticity. Instead, I grew up with this weird, hard-wired toolset for control and image management that became unnecessary and painful, but setting that toolbox down and walking away from it felt like Thor walking away from his hammer, or Captain America putting his shield down for good. Why would I willingly give up what had protected me all my life? Putting Thor's hammer aside was a kind of death. A literal part of myself had to go and it was so central to my being that I couldn't do it on my own.

This knowledge, this awareness, was such a raw moment for me. The Holy Spirit didn't accuse me for the sins of pride, judgment, and unforgiveness. He showed me that these are the things Jesus died for me to overcome. Instead, He took me back to the moment I internalized that Thor's hammer was key to my survival, and supported me while I decided to put it away forever.

Next, like a 12-step program, the Holy Spirit walked me through the garden of weeds that grew from the seeds of abandonment and neglect as a child. I handed the hammer back to Thor, but Jesus was there to take my hand instead, and He promised that He would help me do something about other hurting children, and it would start with my daughter. That I could trust that He sees every child, every situation, that He is there with them and help is on the way.

No way could He have done this early in my battle with illness. I would have collapsed beneath the weight of the walk alone. He had to strengthen me for the walk, but at the end of the garden was a gate, and we walked through that gate together in freedom.

Freedom in this world cannot be defined as the absence of problems, setbacks or attacks. It must be defined as the ability to face problems, setbacks or attacks with the power of God. My garden is still there and the necklace is close at hand. The difference is that now I know what is a weed in my thoughts, and I reach down and pluck it from my garden before it takes root. I can tell when my emotional response to something is based on seeing a person or a situation through a lens on my old necklace and I approach that person, problem or issue with compassion and self-awareness. I still have moments when memories of my failures make me cringe, but I have kindness for myself now and instead of focusing on the pain, I switch my focus around for ways to be good to children; to see, to pray, to support, to provide for children so they can build a better toolbox.

Switching my focus back is as simple as saying, "I forgive X, or myself," and it doesn't matter how I feel as I say it. This is one of the areas where God taking as little as I have to give is so valuable because when I need to forgive someone, I often don't feel like doing it at all. But according to God's Word, it doesn't matter how I feel, it matters what I say and what I offer to Him. So I say out loud that I forgive someone and trust God to do the rest. Listening to a sermon on YouTube, speaking scripture out loud and, especially, worshipping and blessing God and others helps my heaviness to leave, and all the possibilities open up for me again in the space created by focusing on God alone.

Father, please reveal to me any unforgiveness or bitterness that remains in my heart and help me to release it, help me to stay in You every day now as the countdown to the surgery date nears. And Jesus, I'm not going to forget about Your promise to me about helping children. You are my Thor's hammer now, and I am choosing to trust You.

At that point, I could honestly say I felt great, I felt wonderful. Father, glorify Yourself, Thank You for my healing, Thank You for my restoration! Amen and Amen.

DAY 6 OF THE NOVENA OF SURRENDER

I was not thinking or stressing about the upcoming "surgery event," as I considered it. I found that my default was to assume it would happen, so thoughts came up in that vein and I rethought them or replaced them with "I will not have this surgery."

My husband caught a cold and I was getting over it. At my pre-admission testing, they said if it wasn't gone by Wednesday, they would need to reschedule. Is this what you were talking about, God? A reschedule because of a chest cold? It didn't seem like miracle-worthy material, but I was fresh out of my "no judgment" experience, so I chose to go with it.

According to my test results, my blood pressure and heart rate were high, which was not the norm for me. Was I stressing out unconsciously? I didn't think so, I felt at peace about the surgery. When my mind started to head down a road, imagining bad outcomes, I stopped and switched to a worship song in my head or I thanked God for my healing. I was consciously making space for His miracle in my life, keeping my faith up, so I pictured an empty room with light streaming in the windows, waiting with positive expectations, or standing in an open green field, my own Minecraft miracle waiting to be built.

My family thought that, except for the ever-present hat on my head, they had their wife/mom back. I was calm again, laughing and happy, not what you would expect from someone facing major cancer surgery. But I knew the reason was that God was doing a work in my life, in my spirit that was freeing me from so much more than cancer. I was relieved, and I didn't care about the surgery. I felt that it honestly was not my problem, it was God's, and He told me that He had it under control, that it was His battle, not mine. So I operated as if the surgery was not happening, all the while keeping the appointments I was expected to keep, getting my pre-testing, my prescriptions, all the things associated with an upcoming surgery. Odd, I know, but I felt the presence of God covering me hour after hour, day after day.

DAY 6

You are sleepless;
you want to judge everything,
direct everything and see to everything
and you surrender to human strength,
or worse—to men themselves,
trusting in their intervention,
this is what hinders my words and my views.
Oh, how much I wish from you this surrender,
to help you and how I suffer when I see you so agitated!
Satan tries to do exactly this:
to agitate you and to remove you from my protection
and to throw you into the jaws of human initiative.
So, trust only in me,
rest in me,
surrender to me in everything.

Repeat 10 times...

O Jesus, I surrender myself to you,
take care of everything!

This is why I believe God will do what He said:

Against all hope, Abraham in hope believed and so became the father of many nations, just as it had been said to him, "So shall your offspring be." Without weakening in his faith, he faced the fact that his body was as good as dead—since he was about a hundred years old—and that Sarah's womb was also dead. Yet he did not waver through unbelief regarding the promise of God but was strengthened in his faith and gave glory to God, being fully persuaded that God had the power to do what He had promised. This is why "it was credited to him as righteousness." The words "it was credited to him" were written not for him alone, but also for us, to whom God will credit righteousness—for us who believe in him who raised Jesus our Lord from the dead. He was delivered over to death for our sins and was raised to life for our justification.

ROMANS 4:1-23

Abraham was told he would have a son and didn't waver in his belief then, or years later when he was told to sacrifice the son he waited so long to have. And we have the same opportunity to exhibit unwavering faith. I want to know God better and I believe this is one way to do it; by believing what He says.

I felt that believing God, taking Him at His Word, was behavior that would bear fruit, and as I recounted in my mind all the miracles He had done in my life up to that time, I had to admit He was there. I had drawn up a list of everything that concerned me since the day of the biopsy. Every financial thing, every physical thing, everything impacting my family, my friends, my job, whether it was as mundane as filing taxes or being able to attend my daughter's school functions, I wrote it down. And each time something I was concerned about resolved itself, I checked it off the list. And every week I could see progress, I could see my life advancing and it encouraged me. My word at that time was Restoration, and I would pepper my work calendar, notepads, and daily emails with the word. Wherever I could fit the word, I used it. I spoke it out loud over my body and my finances and my life. And of course, one of my daily verses during that time was from the Passion Translation:

I hear Him whisper..."Restoration in 2017"

I will restore you. Do not be afraid to follow me into the unknown, for I am the one who leads you on and restores your life. I have placed within you My glorious treasure, and I care for you. This year will be a year of restoration in your life. You will end this coming year restored in My love, strengthened in My grace, and surrounded with songs of joy. And your joy will be shared by angels, for they are with you, My child, they walk beside you, guarding your life and preparing the way.

I will restore you. Never limit Me. I will restore your family and those you love, they will see Me in your life and know that I am the One who gives back to you what has been lost. Don't doubt My grace that is enough for you and your family.

I say to you, I will restore you and provide for you in ways that will reveal My heart of love. My mercy brings gifts and surprises and supplies all that you need. There will always be provision for your needs, and in My mercy, I will reveal where you can find Me, for this will be the season of abundant supply for every need you have.

I will restore your mind and your heart as you come before Me. Crooked things will be made straight within you. For everything I do for you I do inside your heart, healing your spirit and soothing your soul. Come and find My heart and I will restore your heart. Greater passions will rise within you to feast upon My Word and drink of My Spirit. The hunger I give you will bring you deeper into My grace and My love for you.

I will restore you and your dreams. Those desires within you for completion and to touch the lives of others, I will fulfill. Promises made are promises kept. As I speak deep within you and in the whispers of the night, I will watch over every Word I speak to you and it will be fulfilled.

This day begins a new season of dreams fulfilled. You will laugh with joy when your son of promise, "Isaac" is born. And you will see that My ways are perfect.

PSALM 138:8 THE PASSION TRANSLATION

"You keep every promise you've ever made to me!
Since your love for me is so constant and endless,
I ask you, Lord, to finish every good thing
that you've begun in me!"

25
SURGERY

Surgery was rescheduled for April 4. I have a deep cough and the nurse told me that because of the type of surgery I am having, I would not be able to cough without a great deal of pain, so they would wait one week.

Father, I don't want to have this surgery. I want the doctors to find that there is no cancer anymore and no reason to have it. I want the miraculous to occur, for You to be glorified, for my story to include this encounter with grace.

You won't even let me talk about it. I clam up every time I'm asked about it.

My team at work isn't even aware that surgery is scheduled; that's how sure I am that it won't happen, that Your rhema words to me are about a different kind of challenge.

"You will not have this surgery. Let Me do this for you. Let Me love you, let other people love you. Place no limits on me."

It makes no sense that Your words would apply to that original reschedule. You must have meant them for the whole experience. I quieted my mind and focused on listening for You, but there was no answer, which meant it was up to me, and I chose to believe that You had healed me fully, that I would not have surgery because the cancer was gone.

You were out of the box I always tried to put You in, Lord; not my will but Yours be done. I knew that You wanted me to let go and let You do Your thing.

I surrendered my life, my outcome, and my future and asked You again to please take care of everything.

I was meeting with the surgeons in the afternoon to place a marker inside of me that they would use the next morning for what was supposed to be a double mastectomy.

Today, years later, I can still feel the tension I struggled with those last hours before surgery.

I fought to maintain my peace, because Lord, You said I would not have it and I believed You. You told me to trust You, to place no limits on You, to step into the unknown. That doing what You asked was where growth comes from.

But I knew that the next morning I would have to finally say something (maybe, I would have to say something—honestly, You were the one who said I would not have the surgery, so I thought YOU were the one who was going to be doing or saying something, right?)

My stress level was high, but You said Your children are ALWAYS stressed out when they don't have all the details.

What I learned is that having all the details isn't everything it's cracked up to be.

At the beginning of the process, You told me it wouldn't be that bad and it wasn't. You told me I would hold Victoria's granddaughter and I believe that. And I'm still stressed out. I have talked myself out of what You told me multiple times, and then I remember that You are in control and You told me it would be OK.

During those last hours trying to fall asleep, I was baited, attacked, and felt the force of evil working against me, doing double duty to get me to deny You, to limit my trust.

So maybe another reason You don't share everything is that You know that it makes the enemy double down and, honestly, who needs that?

I was not afraid, but my mind had become a battleground.

I slept very little and prayed over the coming surgery, but I didn't know what to say anymore. I could only thank God for deciding for me.

I surfed the internet, searching words like miracle and healing. This had become a strategy for me; finding and reading random accounts of people whose lives had been radically impacted by God.

I couldn't always summon the right thoughts on my own, but it was powerful to read about the miracles of others and fill my mind with their words and experiences.

In this way, I was fulfilling God's scripture to abide in Him, John 15:7. I began sharing the miracles I found on my blog to encourage others as well. I chose to spread the positive wherever I could to help others and show that there was a consequence to trying to frighten me and destroy my peace.

I read the testimony of a mother of an autistic, nonverbal child who used an iPad to share what he heard God saying to him. He called the communication he had with God his "wisdom words," and in one instance, he defined faith as "picture it done."

I had been picturing my healing as done ever since the diagnosis, picturing myself running and working out hard again, golfing with no impediment in my swing, no pain, pictured myself holding my daughter's granddaughter.

I know that I know that I know that I am well.

You have restored me to a place of greater health than before. I want to live in that knowledge, not go see a doctor who is going to deny it and amass a small army of medical experts, drugs, surgeries, and protocols in opposition to You.

I did not feel sick in the first place. I didn't know anything was wrong until You sent me to the doctor for the mammogram, remember?

So since You sent me, I figured that You had a plan the same way You had a plan with Abraham and Isaac.

While Abraham was walking up the mountain with his son, gathering wood for the fire and preparing the altar, he must have been waiting just like I am. It's nerve-wracking at times, and then You cover me with peace.

Strengthen me, Father, send Your angels to support me and fight on my behalf. Jesus, I would never, ever say that my experience is a microdot of the experience You had when You surrendered Yourself for us. But I can say that I get it, that I'm at my Gethsemane. I am sweating blood over an outcome I can't control and that I don't want to, that I know will turn out badly if I do, that I will forfeit something amazing if I do.

Father, I surrender myself completely to Your will, to Your care. Please take care of everything. Jesus, to say "Thank You" for what You did seems so lame, but it's the only thing to say. Thank You a million times for dying for me, for all of us.

In the middle of my struggle, I was looking for something to listen to in the morning, and I opened a link to a sermon from Joel Osteen titled, "Step into the Unknown."

How do you explain this without God?

Making space for you, Father, making space. Whatever happens, I will love and praise you. While I was in the hospital waiting, I read and reread my psalm for the day, Psalm 121:

I lift up my eyes to the mountains—
where does my help come from?
My help comes from the Lord,
the Maker of heaven and earth.
He will not let your foot slip—
he who watches over you will not slumber;
indeed, he who watches over Israel
will neither slumber nor sleep.
The Lord watches over you—
the Lord is your shade at your right hand;
the sun will not harm you by day,
nor the moon by night.
The Lord will keep you from all harm—
he will watch over your life;
the Lord will watch over your coming and going
both now and forevermore.

26

AWAKE

Woke up cancer and breast free. While I was thankful for the cancer being gone, I was completely weirded out about the surgery. Did I fail in the process of putting no limits on You, at letting You and others love me?

Did I step out on my own instead of letting You do this? Was it the enemy and not You who spoke to me? Did I sin in some way or confess scripture wrongly and mess things up for myself? Help me work through this, Holy Spirit, because no matter the outcome, I trust You. You told me to trust you, to place no limits on You, to let You do this for me. And I know that You are in control and that You told me it would be OK.

Three weeks after the surgery, I vacillated between doubt, frustration, and peace. My chest was numb and I walked around with drainage tubes hanging out of me for 2 weeks, crying every time I checked my incisions in the mirror and saw the war zone that was my upper body. Just before the surgery, I was told that because of swelling, I wouldn't be able to get implants immediately; I would have a device called a spacer inserted in the gap where my breast tissue was. This spacer would have balloon-like mechanisms that would be inflated with water to the size of my implants. When my tissue was healed from the mastectomy, I would return for reconstruction surgery. The spacer had an upper and lower plastic rim that felt like I was carrying a surfboard sideways in my chest. It came equipped with a port to fill the balloons; how that would happen, I could not imagine and had no energy to expend trying.

And in an unexpected twist, the doctor said that likely due to the delay in surgery, cancer had spread beyond the original lymph nodes, so I needed radiation as well. Back on the treadmill I went for what turned out to be the most grueling calendar commitment of my whole treatment. Five weeks, five days a week, forty-five-minute drive each way, fifteen minutes of prep for a grand total of seven minutes of actual treatment. This was moot information, since the bottom line was, I had to clear my calendar and adjust my attitude, once again with no time to luxuriate in things like how I was going to make it work. God's grace was there for me, though, because they just "happened" to have a lunchtime slot available. I jumped on it as a positive sign and held onto that as I listened to what needed to happen to prepare for treatment. It was the start of summer, and I was grateful that the drive each way would happen during warm weather.

I found myself running to His robes again. I was not panicking, just trying to manage the confusion I felt. I needed to internalize that God had something planned, that He had this because I was not the type of girl that would turn against Him because of an outcome I couldn't understand. The Holy Spirit reminded me of that moment during the first weeks of the diagnosis when He asked me which way I was going to go; was my belief so weak that it would collapse under the weight of a setback? I resolved that I would not be the devil's easy target. I would not stop believing because satan fought against me.

As I approached my situation from a position of strength in God and the resolve to believe, the Holy Spirit gave me direction. He showed me that spending time on the why was understandable, but, just as in the case of the initial diagnosis, it wasn't productive and often led me to that vortex of depression that didn't benefit anyone, especially me. Life is a choice, to continue to live, to breathe and believe was also a choice; which way was I going to go?

I chose again to live, to exist as if the choice wasn't a choice but a given. I stayed focused on God and my family and the day before me. My courage and my sanity depended on it. When I strayed from that, when my mind began to imagine other outcomes, it was as if I'd crossed an imaginary line into hell on earth. The message was clear. There was nothing of value for me in that domain of thought, and I had plenty of practice switching my thoughts to other topics. I was not denying the reality of my situation but I was hyper-focused on living, and with a child on summer break, a new client to onboard, and the blessed return of an appetite, my spirit was lifted. It was as if the decision to believe was immediately rewarded with a return to life.

I had phantom pain as if I'd had my breasts amputated, which I guess is what happened. I was puffy with chemically-induced water weight, showing a growth of fuzz on my head but not enough to shed the hat-of-the-day show, and my body looked physically wrecked from the waist up, but I was alive, the sun was shining, and it was warm out. I received my second wind and put on makeup, attempting to match my outfit to the bandana on my head, gamely participating in life. My family and I did not ever allow cancer, cancer surgeries or treatments to stop us from living. We used the demands of life to prove that we chose life, to help us ignore cancer and acknowledge life.

My daughter has no concrete memories of illness in our lives; instead, she had the normal memories of summer vacation, birthday parties and holidays, a few of them with me wearing a beanie on my head. Father, I will always be grateful that you filled us with normal memories of this time in our lives, that we overcame by choosing to live our ordinary, everyday lives.

I learned about ways diet impacted cancer and decided that, if cancer wanted sugar and acidic environments to survive and grow, I was going to do what I could to starve it out by modifying my diet. Nobody should be eating processed sugar anyway. The problem was that American food has processed sugar as a baseline ingredient, but no matter the difficulty, I was going to avoid it as much as possible.

166

Finally, God told me this experience wouldn't be that bad, that I would hold my daughter's granddaughter. I was and am holding Him to that. He told me I would survive this, that cancer would not. I reaffirmed my belief and added Luke 1:45 to my prayers:

Blessed is she who has believed that the Lord's word to her will be fulfilled.

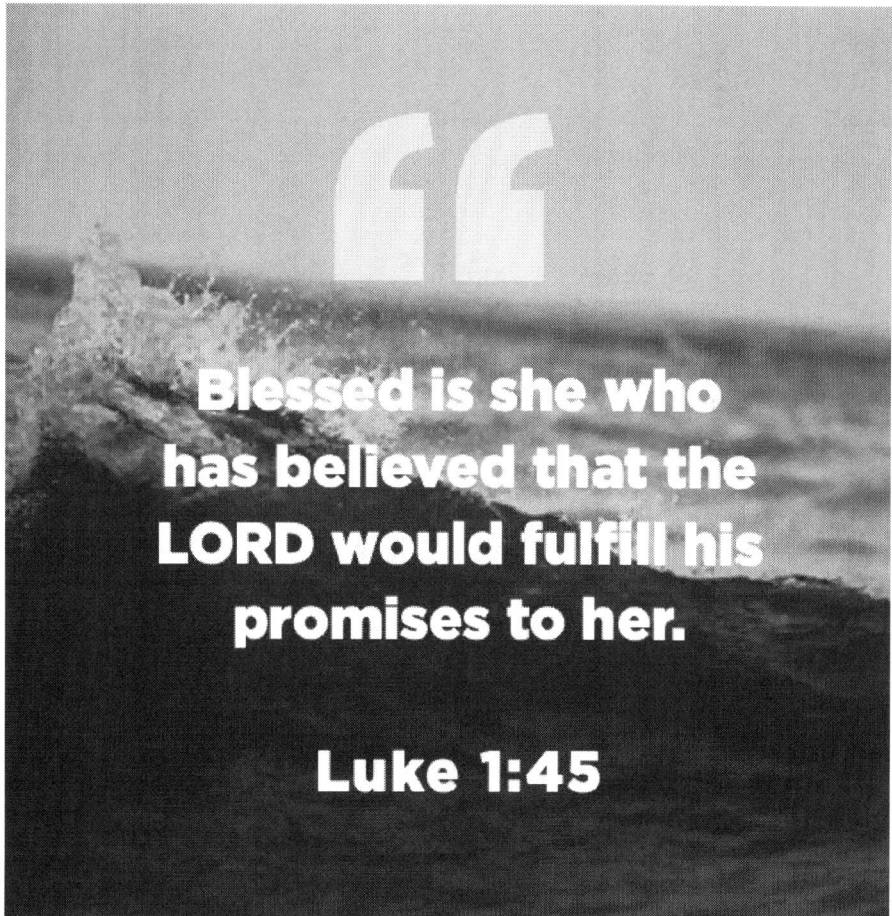

Blessed is she who has believed that the LORD would fulfill his promises to her.

Luke 1:45

My praying friends encouraged me to keep faith with God as well, that He would see my family and me through this time. They reminded me that walking in faith is challenging when we don't get what we think we need, but that's all it is—a challenge. Not a lie, not an exercise in futility, not a denial of reality, just a challenge. And since nothing is impossible with God, and everybody faces challenges every day, I could minimize the scope of my situation in a healthy way and just deal with it. I trusted God would make sense of things. I was certain that He would, so glorify Yourself Father; glorify Yourself.

27

POST SURGERY
TUBES, DRAINS AND DOORKNOBS

Surgery was a combination of a double mastectomy, performed by an oncology surgeon, and preliminary reconstruction done by a plastic surgeon.

They first removed tissue and lymph nodes, inserting surgical drains on either side of my body to drain the fluid from the area the surgeon referred to as "the surgical field," which I interpreted to mean the deflated, hollowed-out place that was once my chest.

The plastic surgeon inserted a hard plate with inflatable balloons called spacers in my chest.

I spent the next two weeks mentally blocking out the experience of draining both sides of my body twice a day like some weird type of dairy cow, and visiting the plastic surgeon to have fluid inserted via a syringe and ports on the spacers to keep room for the implants that would be coming after my tissue healed from the radiation.

I was a human accordion, filling and draining myself every day.

The spacers expanded my chest cavity. It wasn't painful, but it constricted my torso and I would walk around for the next 24 hours with a horse standing on my chest until my body stretched to accommodate the fluid.

Once my skin was stretched out, I would return for another expansion procedure. I understood why the surgeon estimated that it would take two years if I wanted to end up with larger measurements than I went in with.

I couldn't imagine my skin adjusting to a larger size in ten years, let alone two.

I prayed over my body and especially for greater agility. The drains were long tubes that came out of each side of my body and more than once I caught them on a kitchen drawer, or a doorknob.

My husband would hear me yip like a coyote with pain, as I untangled myself, trying not to laugh because that hurt, too. It would seem difficult to feel human during procedures like these, but Father God kept me sane by reminding me that my family needed to know that I was good, that everything would be OK.

A sense of humor and selective memory were key to my progress during this time.

I also developed knob goggles; a sophisticated ability to see protruding doorknobs, drawer pulls and handles of any kind and give them a wide berth.

I imagined myself in heaven with Jesus, many years from now, drinking a glass of red and chewing on a stalk of grass, asking Him the questions that I'd been saving up just for this moment, this one-on-one with Him. And one of the questions will be why, on top of everything else, He allowed the Charlie Chaplin craziness of catching a drainage tube on a doorknob and looking down to check and make sure that my insides were not on my outside. I looked forward to that discussion.

I've been compelled to share many of the most personal experiences I've had on my journey, but some experiences are best left to the imagination.

The process of removing the drainage tubes falls into that category. I praised God for their removal and the immediate block in my memory of the procedure.

Instead, I committed that when I wrote this book I would again share that patients who fight cancer are heroes, and there are millions of them walking around right now; probably within your direct family.

We don't have jackets, but we are members of a world-class club. We don't talk about the battles because that promotes an enemy undeserving of attention.

We don't celebrate the victory often because every single day that we live normally is a victory. But we are thankful, and by the grace of God, who is able, we can be there for others who are fighting.

28

RADIATION

COME GLOW WITH ME

I knew I was fighting a serious illness, but my mind had become so accustomed to the situation that I was mentally fatigued by it.

I couldn't summon the strength to worry, and God didn't want me to anyway. He had strengthened me by surviving chemo and surgery. I felt confident and ready for radiation, even faintly irritated by the necessity of daily appointments 5 days a week for 5 weeks.

There were only two or three things in my life that merited that kind of disciplined focus; my family and my morning devotions.

I didn't feel confident in radiation as a treatment method and prayed hard about protecting my body from the side effects of a form of treatment that could not accurately hit the targeted area with deadly force.

I first had to participate in a prep activity that involved creating temporary tattoos on my chest and back that served as crosshairs for the laser.

While on the table, with my body contorted in awkward poses, I would pray for the precision of the laser aimed at the crosshairs. I would envision the radiation hitting the target, never missing, and all stray cancerous cells being destroyed.

I prayed as Joan Gieson taught me, to see the blood of Christ covering my normal cells, my skin, my lungs, and heart.

I'm a married mom of a nine-year-old who works full time and participates in school sports and activities with friends and family.

Like most American families, mine is busy, whether or not I am sick. As a salesperson, my clients drive my schedule, which means unpredictable things happen regularly.

All of this is to say that I am so grateful that God was dealing out miracles like cards on a blackjack table during those five weeks of radiation.

There were days when I was on a conference call literally up to the point of hopping on the radiation table, but I completed the course of treatment and rang the bell at the end, my daughter by my side.

God is good, all the time. I thanked Him daily for His power over space and time and how He made a way for me so that I was able to keep all my obligations during those highly regimented weeks.

As I neared the end of my 5-week regimen, my main challenge was fatigue. I had been told that I would likely be tired and would need to up my sleep quotient to support healing from the radiation.

I felt strong most of the time, but weariness set in around the third week, and I found myself back on the couch early in the evenings and napping on the weekends.

The sunburn on my skin was minimal, and my discomfort was as well.

I followed all the directions from the nurses, but my Jesus protected my skin so well that I was able to schedule the reconstruction surgery two months ahead of time; a miracle for me, as the spacer in my chest was so uncomfortable. If I twisted to the right or left while bending down, something around the area of my diaphragm would catch on the spacer and I would feel it. It was like having a skateboard-sized plastic spatula in my chest, and I needed it out of my body.

I thanked God for His restoration and prayed that He would cover me while having this final surgery.

29

WHO MOVED MY...

The week before my reconstruction surgery, I received a letter stating that my surgeon was leaving the hospital system, but that he would be able to complete the surgery that I was scheduled to have. I learned that he was scheduled to move out of state the day after my surgery.

I could have viewed this as a huge disappointment, as my surgery follow-ups and future checkups would involve a doctor who was a stranger, but I chose not to dwell on potential problems. In fact, at my pre-op appointment, I learned that he was moving because his wife, also a plastic surgeon, had been offered a leadership position at a hospital elsewhere in the country, and I congratulated them both for her new opportunity.

On the morning of my surgery, my surgeon greeted me and reiterated what would take place. He explained that it would be about an hour and a half to two hours and then I would be on my way home. I had opted for saline implants, which we confirmed, and he headed off to prep.

I waited. And waited. We spoke with the anesthesiologist and my IV was set up. I waited some more. Then my doctor returned, this time in street clothes. He explained that my implants were…missing. But not to worry, as he had located them at another hospital, and was on his way to get them. Since I was his last surgery he didn't want me to be rescheduled with another doctor. So, off he went, in his own car, on his own time, to retrieve my lost implants. Forty-five minutes later he returned, prepped again, and completed my reconstruction.

Some might focus on the unfortunate misplacement of my implants. I focused on the miracle that they were found, that a doctor chose to inconvenience himself for something that was not his fault and that 24 hours from then would not be his problem anyway.

I posted the story of my lost breasts, being driven around Cleveland by a surgeon on his last day of practice in Ohio as a priceless illustration of God's goodness and sense of humor.

I am forever grateful to my surgeon and God for completing my reconstruction surgery, which was also the end of my treatments.

Less than a month later, on my birthday in 2017, my port was removed. Thirteen months after the mammogram that saved my life, my treatments and reconstruction were complete.

During my recovery, the surgeon said something to me that had been mentioned to me throughout all of my treatments—chemo, mastectomy, radiation, and reconstruction—that I "should talk to other patients about my experience," because my attitude was something they rarely saw. But when they did work with someone whose attitude was like mine, the patient survived.

At a complete gut feel, no research whatsoever level of experience, doctors, nurses and other medical professionals shared that the approach the patient took toward their situation was critical to their outcome, and that cancer patients rarely knew how to be optimistic and healing-minded.

The illness struck with such a force of darkness, and the predictability level for recurrence was so sketchy that medical professionals had low confidence in their own ability to heal, it seemed they took a position of, "this is what we know to do, but we guarantee nothing. If you want to survive this illness, you must do something, but we honestly don't know what. Just....something."

In a profession where I had personally witnessed practitioners taking full credit for being absolute experts regarding other illnesses, cancer had become a field where outcomes for healing included patient responsibility, not because of specific health behaviors that needed to be owned by the individual, but because the medical community couldn't own the cure. It was clear why people died from cancer, but they didn't know why some survived.

That's when I heard the Holy Spirit tell me that my experience would help others, that my whole experience, even the part where I thought I would be completely healed without surgery and radiation, would be valuable to people faced with the same confounding illness. That they, like me, would be trying to carve out their unique path to healing like I did, basically taking a machete to the jungle that was my medical crisis.

But maybe my machete left a trail of insights or activities or challenges and battle plans that could lift the cloud of darkness and reveal a path; something that could guide them out of the dark.

I resolved to share everything I could, help in any way I could, to provide support to those who were still fighting. Because the key, I realized, was that cancer is an illness that was about a journey.

My faith accorded me the ability to treat it like a journey, a temporary existence, an adventure I didn't ask for, that nobody asks for but some get regardless.

In the book *World War Z*, the solution that stopped the spread of zombies was a vaccine that rendered those vaccinated imperfect and therefore unattractive to the zombie nation. That's the kind of solution I wanted to see, something simple, scalable, easy to communicate, understand and execute.

But cancer was an individual battle that engaged with me on multiple levels. There was nothing, I repeat, nothing I could do to beat it on my own. My battle against cancer required all hands on deck; the immediate availability of every resource possible to fight.

The aggressiveness of cancer, its ability to morph, regroup, and come back stronger, suggested to me that if I just took it at face value, as a battle against the illness itself, I would not only lose, but I would lose a great deal through the depletion of my resources and increase in the accumulation of negative experiences from treatments that were extended medical torture.

What could pose such a multi-faceted yet perfectly targeted physical threat? What if this illness, whose defining characteristic is to grow like mad, to fight to grow, to return after ridiculous attempts to stop it from growing, is really just my body attempting to do something it thinks it's supposed to do?

The strong sense I had, the battle position that continued to grow as feasible in my mind, as well as resonating with my spirit, was that my cells thought there was an endgame to their growth. And that end game was so real, so attractive to them, that their intelligence at the cellular level was working brilliantly to win the battle and grow like crazy.

Whenever I had an odd ache or heard the story of someone whose cancer returned two, three, five, ten years later with a virulence that was astounding, I would stop and converse with myself, informing my body that the urge to grow like mad was a lie. It was a trick to drive my body to destroy itself, and that the only thing that would happen once my cells were free to grow to their content was their death. It was inevitable because I was, I am, the host, and without me, their growth stops. That we are doing things together now, we are growing as a body and doing things, and nothing required that they get hepped up and start dividing like a colony of insane bunnies.

Does it work? I don't know, but I choose to think that it does because it's hard enough to fight cancer into remission; it shouldn't require that I remain cancer-free for forty years to claim victory.

My victory is now, it's today, and I am creating in real life so my cells don't have to create without my consent.

30
GIVE A BODY A BREAK

I had gained over 20 pounds, much of which appeared to be fluid retention as my organs worked to detoxify my system from the chemical assault by chemo, anesthesia, and radiation. Coupled with total hair loss and a fitness level that plummeted to below that of a sloth in a coma and you had me, but I was determined it would not be for long. It was getting warmer out, and I started getting out on the bicycle every day.

The first two days on the bike, I fell off. As in, I plunged off my bike and had to call my husband to come with the truck to pick the bike and me up and return home. Fell. Both. Days. It was as if my overall body strength had been zapped; I hadn't fallen off a bicycle since I was 8 years old; the prior year I had ridden 20 miles at a time on my bike, but I was weak and quickly winded.

My husband picked me up both times, fixed the chain on my gears and made sure he was around every day for the next two weeks as I ventured out again. I didn't care about the falls, they seemed to happen in slow motion and I wasn't hurt at all. I prayed protection over my body as I regained my strength and thanked God for my restoration, for my healing, and my husband. Each day I got a little farther every day and gained strength.

Just to round out the whole experience for me, I gained 20 pounds without the actual pleasure of eating 20 pounds worth of bakery, or ice cream or alfredo sauce. I could research exactly why this happened, but I wouldn't give cancer that kind of airtime in my life; the bottom line was that, through a combination of increased exercise and decrease in calories, I needed to lose the weight, pronto. I made a meal plan and continued my baby steps approach to cardio training; I didn't feel ready to return to weight training yet.

Many foods made in America have ingredients that are some form of sugar, and highly processed foods can be sugar mixed with chemicals. My diet changed as food became less important to me as an emotional comfort; it took months before the sight of food stopped inducing nausea – today I still tend to jump up first from the dinner table. That makes eating fewer calories easier but those calories now have to come from raw or as close to raw as possible. I chose to balance my pH through my water, offset acidity with apple cider vinegar in my diet, strictly limit carbohydrates and say no to food with ingredients that totaled more than 4 or 5 items.

Raw food only, stay away from sugar and processed foods, limit carbs, exercise every day. Simple plan. But every day, my body wanted to do exactly the opposite. It wanted to sleep, and then tuck into some waffles with nitrate-laden breakfast sausage, then back to sleep. Every day I chose and I tried to choose wisely; some days I was wiser than others. It would be another year before my body was strong and rested again.

A friend of mine, who is a survivor of two-stage four episodes, reminded me that cancer is a huge mind game; knowing that is half the battle. As I forced myself to move when I wanted to rest; to eat my way through mandarin sliced raw Brussels sprouts, to douse the scars on my body with healing oil; I agreed with him; I knew it was a mind game and shared how I viewed it as creation gone awry at the cellular level. We agreed that it is a game that has already been lost by satan, but it's an area that he's been successful in the steal/kill/destroy department and he's not giving up easy.

My nearly bald head shocked me every time I looked in the mirror, but I could see enough fuzz now to look like maybe my style was actually a style, so I wore it proudly.

Now the time has passed; I'm not in chemo, the cancer is gone, my bills are paid, my family is happy again. I suffer a lingering PTSD that is overcome by prayer, by thanking God and calling to Jesus, but if this is all that remains of my experience, I am incredibly fortunate, and I want to share that fortune with others; with everyone who feels drawn to this story.

The question I'm asked most often is about having surgery – about why it happened when God told me that it wouldn't. For now, my answer is twofold. First, I don't doubt God's word to me. In Proverbs 30:5 it says, "Every word of God is pure. He is a shield unto them that put their trust in Him." I wait in faith to understand what His words meant to me. Like Abraham waited as he walked his only son to the altar, or Moses waited at the shore of the Red Sea with the Egyptian army bearing down on him. People who believe God have waited for weirder things, that's for sure. Joshua walking around Jericho for the fourth time; what could he have been thinking? So I have joined the ranks of those who wait on the Lord and count my blessings.

Second, by giving me those words, He set my feet on a path and gave me a mission for my life. To seek Him in order to learn more about Him and to share what I learn with others. To be caught in His web of miracles and charged with showing others what He's capable of; what He's about. It's a divine adventure and I'm honored to follow this path with Him, because He will never leave me nor forsake me (Deut. 31:6).

I listen to Bill Winston while I'm riding; I know whose I am; who I belong to; I'm a full mantle wearing, covenant bearing, Christ declaring daughter of Abraham; performing signs, wonders and miracles because Jesus, MY JESUS, went to be with the Father. My purpose now, my mission, is to care for my family and my ministries; to serve God by healing the sick, and teaching others to do the same; to glorify God and witness to His miracles and the wonders He does for men.

THESE PRAYERS ARE FOR YOU!

HEALING PROPHECY

Father, I know You are prophesying over my life now and I add to this prophecy my thanks and gratitude to You for the blessings You have poured out on my life, even though others looking at my life right now might think the opposite. My testimony doesn't come from the final victory alone, it also comes from the faith that allowed me to stand when everything was coming against me. It comes from the incredible experience of being loved by You through a difficult situation and being introduced to people that You sent to surround me so that I would know Your care during this frightening, looking-death-in-the-eye season. I will forever be grateful for the closeness we share right now. In the name of Jesus Christ of Nazareth, I declare healing over my body; I declare that I am completely healed from cancer, cancer treatments, and surgeries. My body is operating in love, in the fullness of Christ, and as God intended it. In Jesus's name, Amen.

LIFE AFFIRMATION

Jesus said, "No one takes it (my life) from me, but I lay it down of my own accord. I have authority to lay it down and authority to take it up again. This command I received from my Father." I take this as a command for me as well, and I declare now that I do not now and never will lay my life down for cancer, cancer treatments, or side effects of cancer. I will not lay my life down for any accidents, illness, injury, sickness or disease. I will not lay my life down for any attacks or demons coming against me. I do not lay my life down for another 60 years at least. And should Jesus, my Jesus, return during that time, I will be able to answer YES when He asks, "Is there still faith on the earth?" Amen.

DECLARATION OF HEALING

In the name of the Lord Jesus Christ of Nazareth, I declare that all cancer, side effects from cancer, cancer treatments, and surgeries leave me now; that Jesus Himself is restoring my body and that it now operates as God intended it. By the power of Jesus, who took all sickness and disease with Him to the cross and left it there, I declare I am healed of cancer, all cancer side effects, and all fear and anxiety.

In Christ Jesus, who makes all things new, I declare that all the cells in my body are aligning with the Word of God and operating as they were originally designed. I command all the cells in my body that were negatively impacted by cancer, cancer side effects, fear and anxiety to line up with God's Truth that I am fearfully and wonderfully made. Holy Spirit, please destroy all cells that refuse to change to accept God's Truth. I speak to every generation of cells in my body and call forth the creation of new, strong, powerful and healthy cells. I bless them with the abundant life of the Lord Jesus Christ! Thank you, Father!

HEALING FOR OTHERS FIGHTING CANCER

In the name of Jesus, I (we) command that (person's name) cancer be destroyed at the root, never to return, that the root of cancer in (person's name) body leave now, in the name of Jesus. I declare in Jesus's name that all cancer and side effects of cancer and cancer treatments will never harm (person's name). I command that (person's name) DNA, their body chemistry and genetics change now to conform to God's original intention, His original design for them. I declare that Jesus is restoring to (person's name) everything they lost, and He always restores to a place greater than before; so now (person's name) has greater health, greater well-being, and wellness. In Jesus's name. Amen.

SEVENFOLD RESTORATION

In the name of Jesus Christ of Nazareth, I declare satan has been stealing my peace and my health, along with the health of millions of people fighting cancer. The word of the Lord in Proverbs 6:31 states, "yet if he is caught, he must pay sevenfold, though it costs him all the wealth of his house." I declare satan has been caught and he is now paying me along with everyone that is fighting cancer back sevenfold for everything stolen from us all. Amen.

PRAYERS TO OVERCOME FEAR

And now, we break the assignment of the enemy to continuously afflict me with loss and fear. And I declare in the name of Jesus Christ of Nazareth whom I serve, that all trauma, all lack of any kind, all illness, infirmity, accident, injury or attack LEAVES NOW. And Jesus Himself restores what has been stolen from me. Jesus is the God of restoration, and He always restores to a place that is greater than before, therefor I now possess greater health, greater spiritual growth, greater abundance, greater security. Thank you for my restoration Lord. Thank you for my healing.

Made in the USA
Columbia, SC
25 August 2022